Eat Fat and Get Thin, Fit, and Healthier Than Ever Before!

Easy Diet and Delicious Cookbook: Recipes for Dramatic and Sustainable Weight Loss (Includes 21 Day Meal Plan)

By: Robert Roma

Eat Fat and Get Thin, Fit, and Healthier Than Ever Before!

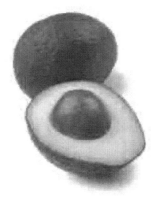

Eat Fat and Get Thin, Fit, and Healthier Than Ever Before!

Legal notice

Table of Contents

Eat Fat and Get Thin, Fit, and Healthier Than Ever Before!

Eat Fat and Get Thin, Fit, and Healthier Than Ever Before!

This book is divided into three parts. The first part of the book explains the truth about consuming fats. This explanation aims to be scientifically sound while still remaining accessible to readers of any background. By the end of this section, you will understand which fats are healthy, how they impact your health, as well as the mistakes, lies, and dirty secrets that have led to our current state of mass confusion about fat consumption.

The second part of this book is a cookbook. It is loaded with dozens of tasty and delicious recipes you will want to eat again and again. The recipes require no exotic equipment or expert cooking background. They may look like a million bucks on your plate, but most of the recipes in this book can be made for only a few dollars per plate. Most importantly, each and every recipe you will find in this book is informed by a simple truth that you will fully understand by the time you are finished reading this book: if you want to get thin, fit, and healthy, you need to eat fat!

Finally, the third part of this book is a complete 21 day meal plan. The meal plan provides a delicious breakfast, lunch, and dinner you can prepare for yourself alone or for your entire family every day for 21 days. The meals are so delicious you won't even realize you are on a diet. Before you begin the 21 day meal plan take a moment to weigh yourself. Check your weight again after completing the 21 day meal plan and you will see for yourself that you can lose a significant amount of weight just by eating delicious, healthy fat!

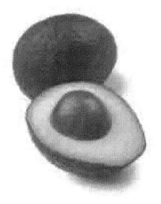

Part 1: The Skinny on Fat

Introduction

Before we can have an informed discussion about the role fat plays in a healthy diet, we need to set down some basic distinctions between the various kinds of fats that exist. There are many different kinds of fat and each type can impact your health in different ways.

Fats are responsible for many healthy functions in the body. Fats store energy, coat membranes, insulate tissues, and protect vital organs. You may have heard the term "lipid" before when reading about the topic of fat. The term "lipid" refers to a group of hydrocarbons (a string of carbon atoms surrounded by hydrogen atoms). This group includes all fats and many other basic molecules that exist in the body. For example, cholesterol, triglycerides, and certain vitamins such as A, D, E, and K, are all lipids. Despite their similarities, different sources of fat form different chains of atoms and are processed by your body in different ways.

The three lipids we typically hear about when it comes to food are saturated fats, unsaturated fats, and trans fats. It isn't necessary for our purposes to dive into the specific atomic differences that exist between the various kinds of lipids – don't worry, this isn't an organic chemistry textbook. What matters here is how these different types of fat impact your health and weight when they are consumed.

What you will learn in this book may surprise you, but by the time you reach the end you will understand why fat is not the demon it has been made out to be. Quite the opposite. In fact, eating fat is an essential part of losing weight, getting thin and fit,

Eat Fat and Get Thin, Fit, and Healthier Than Ever Before!

and living a healthy life.

The Calorie Myth

It is practically considered gospel truth to nutritionists and the medical profession alike that people who consume more calories than they burn will get fat. They believe that the obesity epidemic facing the Western world today is caused by people eating too many calories and not being active enough. It would be easy to believe that fat people are just idle and indulgent, but this is a myth.

Perhaps the most obvious problem with this theory is that it fails to explain why some people regularly consume more calories than they actually need without ever getting fat. Further, many cases have shown that even *underfed* people can get fat. There are various examples throughout history where those living in poverty were actually the most overweight. This certainly didn't come about as a result of an abundance of food!

Another obvious problem for this flawed but popular theory is that it is silent on how it is possible for two people with similar lifestyles to have significantly different body fat profiles. Anyone seriously interested in losing weight needs to question this often unexamined edict of modern nutrition science.

A further problem with the theory that too many calories and too little exercise causes obesity is that when you exercise more, your body *requires* that you consume more calories to function. This boosts our appetite and causes us to eat more. Perhaps surprisingly, there is actually very little evidence that exercise alone prevents obesity.

The Dawn of an Error

Roughly half a century ago a new idea came into vogue and has been popular ever since. This idea is that consuming fat is what makes us fat. Doctors, nutritionists, and the FDA took up the charge, warning people of the detrimental effects consuming fat can have on our bodies and our health. Major food producers got on board too, touting their "fat-free" and "low fat" processed foods, where natural fats were typically replaced with simple carbohydrates like flour or sugar, or impressive lists of chemicals that don't sound like anything your grandmother would have cooked with.

The fact is that eating less and exercising more is not what prevents us from being overweight, despite the fact that these two things are typically used to explain obesity. What really matters is not how much we eat, but rather *what kind* of food we eat, and especially *how those foods impact our insulin levels.*

The Crucial Role of Insulin

Insulin is the main culprit behind obesity. This is a key point to understand in the battle against obesity. Further, realize that it is carbohydrates that primarily influence the production of insulin in the body.

The hormone insulin is how our bodies react to the consumption and digestion of carbohydrates. Insulin plays a massively important role in our metabolism because it is responsible for the recycling of all macro nutrients that provide our body with energy. Insulin facilitates the transfer of energy into the muscle tissue where it is burned. It also stimulates our fatty tissue to store extra energy that we don't need. Storing extra energy that we don't need is another way of saying "getting fat". When we eat a meal, our bodies want to deal with that energy immediately. And as soon as carbohydrates hit our bloodstream in the form of glucose, our blood-sugar level spikes. High blood-sugar levels can cause an adverse reaction to a variety of cells, which means the body wants to regulate the blood-sugar level quickly. It does this by using hormones and by quickly burning up the energy that can most easily be used as fuel. The flood of insulin in the body marks the beginning of this process. The amount of insulin that gets released is dependent on the quantity of carbohydrates consumed and absorbed. Excess energy, regardless of its macro nutrient source, is stored as fat for later use. Food rich in carbohydrates stimulates this insulin release. The more carbohydrates, the more insulin is released. The more insulin released, the more our body works to store fat. This is how we *really* get fat.

HOW CARBOHYDRATE CONSUMPTION CAUSES FAT STORAGE

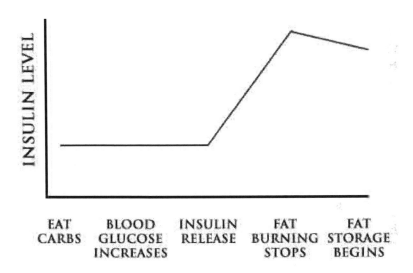

Processing popular modern carbohydrates

Humans really are creatures of habit. Throughout most of human history our diets were fairly consistent. What humans ate for most of the time we've existed on Earth is not the highly processed, refined carbohydrate foods we eat today. Although humans have inhabited Earth for something like 2.5 million years, we have been consuming flour for only a small fraction of that. White flour and sugar only became a significant part of the human diet towards the end of the 19th century. It is inconceivable that we have genetically adapted to our radical new diets in such a short period of time. Our ancestors consumed diets consisting of lots of fish, meat, fat, and protein. Many survived without eating fruit or grains at all.

Carbohydrates make us sick

Long-term consumption of large quantities of carbohydrates can throw-off the delicate mechanism that determines when and how much insulin to release. The result is that we end up with too much insulin. This is problematic. First of all it makes us fat, but second of all it erodes our health and exposes us to certain risks and chronic diseases like diabetes and high blood-sugar. These are diseases often thought of as being caused by obesity. In fact they are actually a symptom of excessive carbohydrate consumption, just as obesity itself is as well! This is why these diseases suddenly take hold in populations first exposed to Western diets, as well as new immigrants to the West. Demonizing the entire Western lifestyle is throwing the baby out with the bath water. It is not our lifestyle that is the problem. The problem is excessive carbohydrate consumption and inadequate fat consumption!

Low calorie diets are ineffective and dangerous

Low calorie diets can be effective in the short term, but they rarely work in the long term. This is because low calorie diets restrict our consumption of the energy our bodies need to be fit and healthy. These diets literally starve our bodies, and although we may lose weight when we are on them, as soon as we're off them we have a tendency to boomerang right back to where our body weight was before, or worse! Studies have shown that low calorie diets, even when they contain high nutrient foods and little fat, rarely lead to much weight loss. Further, some studies have actually shown that a majority of the weight lost by "low calorie" dieters is actually weight from muscle and not fat!

What other factors contribute to obesity?

One way we can combat fat storage is by reducing our intake of carbohydrates. This is not the whole story however. Our genes determine both how quickly we store energy, where we store it, and how quickly we can burn it off later. Some people are more prone to being fat, while others can eat two helpings of desert without ever becoming obese. Also, the levels of insulin we generate and release can change over time. When we routinely release insulin our body can become "insulin resistant", meaning our bodies are inhibited from burning energy. The body reacts by releasing more and more insulin in order to lower our blood sugar. This only strengthens the resistance and encourages the growth of fat cells. Insulin resistance often increases with age, which is why older people are more prone to be overweight. It is not a matter of one's metabolism "slowing down", but rather it is a lifetime of eating carbohydrates and building insulin resistance that causes this. Fortunately, there is hope for anyone, even those who are disadvantaged by "bad" genes, or folks who have subsisted for decades on processed, sugary, high carbohydrate junk food. By committing to a healthy high fat diet today, you can slowly but surely overcome those obstacles to good health.

The Deadly Secrets of the Sugar Industry

There has been evidence linking sugar to a myriad of deadly, chronic diseases for at least half a century. Think about that for a moment. *Deadly* chronic diseases. It is not hyperbole to say that sugar kills. There is ample scientific evidence for it, and yet it seems to go unnoticed and ignored by the general public, the food industry, and government regulators alike. Why is that? How can it be that the *scientific fact* that sugar is deadly is not also a well known fact? How can it be that sugar is so ubiquitous in the products that line grocery store shelves? How can it possibly be, that with all of this evidence, the food industry blissfully fills boxes of cereal with industrial strength quantities of sugar and then markets them *directly at young children?!* If this were virtually any other product and any other industry, this practice would have ceased a very long time ago as soon as the evidence became clear.

The reason why all these things continue to this day is one of the dirtiest, deadliest secrets of the sugar industry. Compelling documentation exists that invites us to draw the conclusion that the sugar industry has waged a decades long war against the popularization of scientific fact. This evidence takes the form of internal newsletters, government lobbying, speeches and presentations given to select groups of influential people, etc. The campaign that has been waged by the sugar industry over the last half a century is similar to the efforts of the tobacco industry to keep the link between their products and cancer rates under wraps.

Sugar Mountain

The average American consumes almost *80 pounds* of sugar per year. That is a pretty remarkable statistic given the serious and even deadly harm caused by sugar. The scientific link between sugar consumption and diabetes is 100% conclusive, and yet the machine that is the sugar industry grinds ever onward, chewing up our longevity and quality of life right along with it.

Make no mistake, I'm not claiming that no one is aware sugar is unhealthy. We are all aware of this. But what most people are unaware of is just *how bad* sugar really is for our health. The reason for this has to do with the prevailing myths about what is and is not good for us. We have been led to believe, quite deliberately, that too much fat is the problem with our modern diets. The demonization of fat over the last several decades has opened the door for the rise in consumption of refined carbohydrates like sugar. In the minds of the general public, the words "low fat" on a grocery store product means it is healthy to eat. What it *really* means in many cases is that instead of fat, it is loaded with sugar and other refined carbohydrates that *are actually more likely to make you fat.* This is the obfuscation that has led to our current mass state of delusion and has kept us in the dark about the deadly secret the sugar industry doesn't want anyone to know. The sugar industry is quite content to take that secret all the way to *your* grave.

Does Saturated Fat Cause Heart Disease?

Part of the reason the sugar industry has been so successful in their obfuscation efforts is because it has been accepted as something akin to gospel truth that saturated fat is a cause of heart disease. Heart disease is a leading killer in Western countries and so, if true, this would be an excellent reason to avoid saturated fat in your diet and to eat foods labeled "low fat" instead. But does saturated fat really cause heart disease? When you take a hard look at the scientific data that exists today, there is good reason to be believe otherwise.

One of the reasons why so many people make the assumption that saturated fat causes heart disease is because many of the available studies support that hypothesis. But to get at the truth, we need more than just *support* for that hypothesis, because there can be confounding factors and outside influences that are a part of these studies that may be explained in some other way.

It is easy to become a victim of conventional wisdom however, even for well-meaning scientists. When something is widely believed, rightly or wrongly, there is a tendency to minimize conflicting data points and focus on some other aspect of a study that comports with majority opinion. This is something that occurs very frequently in scientific journals.

I realize that claiming saturated fat does not cause heart disease is very much going against the grain. For the sake of our health, we must challenge this conventional wisdom however, so let's get a little bit more detailed in the explanation of why so many people believe that saturated fat causes heart disease and why this is wrong, despite the hypothesis appearing to have strong scientific support.

What Science Says About Saturated Fat and Heart Disease

There have been several studies that show when you replace some percentage of saturated fat with polyunsaturated fats (these are essential fatty acids like Omega 3 and Omega 6, sometimes colloquially called "healthy fats"), there is a slight improvement in cardiovascular health, including markers like cholesterol, and a slight reduction of certain risks such as heart attacks and strokes. For a lot of people, even smart and well trained scientists, these studies will serve as the basis for their conclusion that saturated fats can cause heart disease and other cardiovascular problems.

The reason why such a conclusion is *not* justified by the evidence is that when you start replacing saturated fats with other things, for example carbohydrates, guess what happens to your risk of heart disease? The *best case* scenario is that your risk remains the same. More often, the evidence shows that your risk actually goes up! Let me say that again: legitimate, peer-reviewed, scientific studies have consistently shown that *removing* saturated fats from a person's diet and replacing them with carbohydrates *increases* that person's risk of heart disease. This strongly suggests that reducing saturated fat intake is not good for our health. It also suggests that based on the studies covered so far, we are not in a position to say anything at all about saturated fat on its own. We can say something about saturated fat relative to polyunsaturated fat: saturated fat is less healthy. We can also say something about saturated fat relative to carbohydrates: saturated fat is more healthy.

This explains the myth that saturated fat is linked to heart disease. The truth is simply that saturated fat is more likely to cause heart disease than "healthy" polyunsaturated fats, but less likely to cause heart disease than carbohydrates. The practical takeaway here is that to promote heart health, you are better off cutting back on carbohydrates and eating more fat.

Are All Carbs Bad?

There is an increasingly popular backlash to the conventional wisdom that is gaining some steam these days in the form of "low carb" or "ketogenic" diets that attempt to greatly restrict or almost entirely eliminate the consumption of carbohydrates. So are all carbohydrates bad for us?

The answer is no, not *all* carbs are bad. Vegetables are mostly carbohydrates, and surely no one is arguing that vegetables are unhealthy. Intact grains have been consistently shown to be healthy as well. So how do we separate the good carbohydrates from the bad carbohydrates and avoid throwing the baby out with the bathwater?

The key to understanding what is really going on with our health and our waistlines when it comes to consuming carbohydrates requires separating carbohydrates that come from natural whole foods (like fruits, vegetables, and intact grains) from carbohydrates that come from foods that have been refined and processed, like sugar.

Some of the early recommendations about *added* sugar (meaning sugars other than those that occur naturally, such as in most fruit) were based on the assumption that sugar was not harmful. This formed a cornerstone of the prevailing dietary recommendations that continues to inform American public policy on the food industry to this day.

The bottom line when it comes to carbohydrates is that the more refined they are, the worse they are for you – and none more so than sugar. Ultimately, whether you choose to eat sugar or abstain completely is up to you, and I certainly don't intend to preach wildly against the dangers of ever having a slice of cake to celebrate one's birthday. My point when it comes to sugar is simply this: it is deadly. Tasty, but deadly. If you are going to consume sugar regularly, or in the quantities that a typical American does, be aware that you are asking for serious health trouble. Be aware also that sugar and other refined carbohydrates are far, far worse for you than fat has ever been.

What About Trans Fats?

Trans fats have gotten a lot of negative attention recently and it is well deserved. The topic of trans fats can be dealt with simply and quickly: trans fats are unhealthy. Do not consume trans fats. No quantity of trans fats will promote or improve your health, and the optimal quantity of trans fats to consume is none at all.

Trans fats became popular in the 1950s when processed foods were relatively new and very much in vogue. Major food companies began industrially engineering vegetable fats to be used in a myriad of food products such as margarine, processed snacks, and fast food. In the last half a century, trans fats have been conclusively linked to obesity, heart attacks, cancer, strokes, inflammation, diabetes, lower rates of good cholesterol, and higher rates of bad cholesterol.

The only good thing that can be said about trans fats is that they are on the way out. The FDA and other government regulators have gotten serious about crafting legislation and public health policy to eliminate the consumption of trans fats. The fact that the trans fat lobbyists have not enjoyed the same level of success as the sugar industry speaks to just how horrible trans fats are for your health!

There is one more insidious fact you should know about trans fats, however. A product that says "no trans fat" on its label may still contain trans fats! If you read the label and see that it contains "partially hydrogenated fat", that product contains trans fat. The reason food manufacturers continue to get away with this is by exploiting a loophole in food labeling guidelines. If a product contains less than half a gram of trans fats per serving, it is legal in many states and countries to label that product as being "trans fat free" or containing "0 trans fats". If you are purchasing a processed food product, be vigilant. Check the label for the word "hydrogenated" and if you see it, leave that product on the shelf!

How to Eat Fat and Get Thin, Fit, and Healthy

As you have seen in the preceding chapters, our fundamental understanding of obesity is totally incorrect. This is the reality that we live in today, and it is past time that we underwent a major paradigm shift in the way we think about health, obesity, and weight loss.

Insulin resistance and obesity have demonstrated links to a shockingly wide variety of chronic disease, including type 2 diabetes, fatty liver disease, stroke, hypertension, sleep apnea, cancer, asthma, Alzheimer's, osteoarthritis, gall bladder disease, and many, many more. What all of these diseases add up to is a reduction in quality of life and longevity.

The things making us overweight are the same things making us sick. Conventional wisdom about obesity is based largely on calorie consumption and the idea that a calorie surplus causes obesity while a calorie deficit causes weight loss. As discussed in the *Calorie Myth* chapter, this is not at all a full account of the issue.

The fact is that nutrition research, education, and beliefs have been almost irredeemably flawed for decades now. Looking at the state of the Western world today, this shouldn't be much of a surprise. If we *really* understood what makes us fat, we would not have the troubling obesity rates that we currently have. Likewise, if we *really* understood what makes us healthy, our rates of chronic disease would be going down, not getting worse.

One of the fascinating things you find when you start to dig into the research that exists on nutrition and public health is that you can find civilizations in the past that have had very high rates of obesity – similar to, or even worse, than what we experience today in the modern world. But these societies didn't have the easy access to processed food that we have today. There wasn't a McDonald's on every corner or a Dunkin' Donuts Drivethru on the way to work. These societies weren't sedentary like ours either. The obese people from these civilizations didn't sit on a chair all day working on a computer because computers hadn't been invented yet. And yet these civilizations that existed in all corners of the globe, from South America, to Africa, to Asia; that lived decades or sometimes even centuries ago, had seriously high rates of obesity. Further, many of these civilizations were extremely poor. They weren't gorging endlessly on food like gluttons because they were living in poverty.

So what is going on here? These civilizations didn't have to deal with the trappings of our stressful modern lives. They lived in a world that was not full of an infinite supply of cheap calories. So why were they so fat? They were physically active, they barely ate enough to survive, and yet they were fat. Why?!?!

The missing link in our understanding of obesity and health is insulin. Insulin secretion and insulin resistance is directly connected to fat storage and fat loss, and yet insulin is so often left completely out of the conversation when it comes to obesity and weight loss. The evidence that establishes insulin as the fundamental regulator of fat metabolism is robust and has been conclusive since the 1960s. If you want to get fat out of the fat cells – in other words, if you want to reduce the amount of stored fat in the body and lose weight – you simply need to get your insulin down. The way you do this is by replacing carbohydrates in your diet with fat. This works because fat is the one nutrient that does not stimulate insulin production and release.

The reason why this *fact* that eating fat promotes weight loss is not well known today is due to some of the reasons discussed above. In the 1960s, erroneous conclusions were being drawn by well-meaning scientists regarding the supposed connection between saturated fat consumption and heart disease. Then there was the deliberate misinformation campaign successfully waged by the sugar industry that has influenced the FDA, public health policy, nutrition labeling, education, and the general understanding of the public about health and the cause of obesity. It was the combination of these factors that caused our collective misunderstanding about heath and obesity, and allowed these misunderstandings to persist to this day.

It is time to dispense with the popular but baseless beliefs about fat. *Consuming fat does not make us fat.* The key to good health and weight loss is eliminating poor and mediocre quality carbohydrates from our diet and replacing them with fat.

Eat Fat and Get Thin, Fit, and Healthier Than Ever Before!

Eat Fat and Get Thin, Fit, and Healthier Than Ever Before!

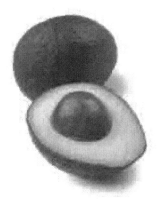

Part 2: Healthy High Fat Recipes

Part 2 of this book is a cookbook full of delicious recipes based on the health and weight loss principles explained in Part 1. There are dozens and dozens of recipes that will suit every taste, every budget, and every skill level in the kitchen. These delicious recipes treat food as the honest and natural source of nutrition that it is. The ingredients are healthy, the methods are not overly complex, and none of the recipes require any exotic equipment or significant cooking background.

By following the principles and recipes in this book, you can lose more weight than you ever thought possible and become fitter and healthier than ever before – all while eating amazing, filling, delicious meals. There is no need to sacrifice tasty food or starve yourself. When you eat fat to get thin, fit, and healthy, you really can have it all!

Breakfast Recipes

White Pizza Frittata

Serves: 8
Time: About 35 minutes

Pizza for breakfast? Absolutely! This keto-friendly pizza is really a frittata, but it uses ingredients usually found in a pizza like pepperoni and mozzarella cheese. Each serving packs a whooping 19.4 grams of protein, 23.8 grams of fat, and only 2.1 carbs.

Ingredients:

12 big eggs
9 ounces of frozen spinach
5 ounces of mozzarella cheese
1 ounce of pepperoni
½ cup of parmesan cheese
½ cup of fresh ricotta cheese
4 tablespoons extra-virgin olive oil
1 teaspoon minced garlic
¼ teaspoon nutmeg
Salt and pepper to taste

Directions:

1. Microwave the frozen spinach for 3-4 minutes.
2. Squeeze to get out as much liquid as possible.

3. Preheat the oven to 375-degrees.

4. Mix the eggs, spices, and olive oil together in a large bowl.

5. Add the ricotta and spinach, using a spatula to break up the greens.

6. Pour into a cast-iron skillet and sprinkle the mozzarella on top.

7. Arrange the pepperoni on top.

8. Bake for 30 minutes.

9. Cool before serving!

Nutritional Info:

Total calories: 298
Carbs: 2.1
Fat: 23.8
Protein: 19.4
Fiber: <1

Breakfast Mug Cake

Serves: 1
Time: About 2 minutes

When you think of mug cakes, you probably think of a dessert, but you can make savory mug cakes, too! This breakfast cake uses a very simple base that includes almond flour, and delicious breakfast goodies like bacon and cheese.

Ingredients:

1 big egg
2 tablespoons almond flour
2 tablespoons butter
2 slices cooked bacon
1 tablespoon almond flour
1 tablespoon shredded cheddar cheese
1 tablespoon shredded white cheddar cheese
1 tablespoon chopped chive
½ teaspoon baking powder
Salt and pepper to taste

Directions:

1. Mix the 2 tablespoons almond flour, baking powder, butter, and egg together.
2. Chop the bacon and chives.
3. Mix everything together in a mug and microwave for 65 seconds on the high setting.
4. To remove the cake, tap the mug upside down on a plate.
5. Season to taste and enjoy!

Nutritional Info:

Total calories: 573
Carbs: 5
Fat: 55
Protein: 24
Fiber: 2

Chicken Sausage Breakfast Pie

Serves: 2-3
Time: About 30 minutes

High in protein and fat, this breakfast pie will leave you feeling satisfied and happy even during the longest mornings. This particular recipe calls for cheddar-and-bacon chicken sausages, but you can use any chicken sausage you would like.

<u>Ingredients:</u>

1 ½ cheddar-and-bacon chicken sausages
¾ cup grated cheddar cheese
5 egg yolks
¼ cup coconut oil
¼ cup coconut flour
2 tablespoons coconut milk
2 teaspoons lemon juice
½ teaspoon rosemary
¼ teaspoon baking soda
¼ teaspoon cayenne pepper
⅛ teaspoon salt

<u>Directions:</u>

1. Preheat your oven to 350-degrees.
2. Cube the chicken sausages and fry over medium-heat
3. Mix the flour and other dry ingredients (including spices) together.
4. Beat the egg yolks for 4-5 minutes before adding the lemon juice, coconut milk, and coconut oil.
5. Mix well.

6. Slowly pour the wet ingredients into the dry.

7. Fold in ½ cup of cheese.

8. Take out 2 ramekins and fill to the ¾ line.

9. Arrange the sausage in the ramekins, so the cubes are evenly-distributed.

10. Bake for 20-25 minutes.

11. Add the rest of the cheese and put under the broil for another 3-4 minutes.

12. Serve!

Nutritional Info (2 servings):

Total calories: 711
Carbs: 5.8
Fat: 65.3
Protein: 34.3
Fiber: 5.8

Jalapeno-Popper Cups

Serves: 12
Time: About 25-30 minutes

When you think of jalapeno poppers, you probably think of bar food, but this recipe lets you eat them for breakfast or a portable snack. You make them in a muffin tin, so they're super convenient.

Ingredients:

12 strips of bacon
8 big eggs
3 medium-sized seeded and chopped jalapeno peppers
1 jalapeno pepper, cut into rings
4 ounces of cheddar cheese
3 ounces of cream cheese
½ teaspoon onion powder
½ teaspoon garlic powder
Salt and pepper to taste

Directions:

1. Preheat your oven to 375-degrees.
2. Cook the bacon, so it's crisp, but you can still bend it without it breaking.
3. Save the bacon grease.
4. Mix the rest of the ingredients (minus the ringed jalapeno pepper and the cheese).
5. Grease the muffin tin and encircle the muffin cups with the bacon.
6. Pour the egg mixture into the cups, about halfway.
7. Sprinkle on the cheese and top with a ring of jalapeno.

8. Cook for 20-25 minutes.
9. Cool before eating.

Nutritional Info:

Total calories: 216
Carbs: .9
Fat: 19.3
Protein: 9.6
Fiber: <1

Fast and Cheesy Jalapeno Cheddar Waffles

Are you on the lookout for a sweet and a savoury treat that you can take as breakfast? Then, look no more for here comes a feisty dish in which cheddar cheese coalesces with jalapeno to make a simple yet tasty dish that can be bought to the table within 15 minutes!

Preparation Time: 8 Minutes
Cooking Time: 7 Minutes
Servings: 2 Servings
Ingredients:

- 3 oz. Cream Cheese

- 1 teaspoon Psyllium Husk Powder

- 3 Eggs, preferably large and organic

- 1 Jalapeno, small

- 1 tablespoon Coconut Flour

- Sea Salt, to taste

- 1 teaspoon Baking Powder

- Pepper, to taste

- 1 oz. Cheddar Cheese

Method of Preparation:

- To start with, combine all the ingredients, excluding the cheese and jalapeno, in a medium sized bowl and blend them with the help of an immersion blender. (Tip: if you don't have an immersion blender, you can mix them together in a food processor.)

- Once it is well incorporated, stir in the cheese and the jalapeno into the bowl and mix them again using the immersion blender until they are properly blended.

- After that, heat the waffle iron and once it is hot, pour the batter into it and cook for about five to six minutes or until it is cooked and golden yellow in colour.

- Then, remove the waffles from the waffle iron and transfer them to the serving plate.

- Finally, top it with the choice of your toppings and enjoy your savoury breakfast.

Tip: It pairs well with avocado and full-fat sour cream.

Nutritional Information:
➢ Calories – 338 kcal
➢ Fat – 28gm
➢ Carbohydrates – 3gm
➢ Protein – 16gm
➢ Fiber – 3gm

Green Eggs and Butter

What makes this simple dish different from the other usual breakfast fares is the robust flavour that comes through this nutritious dish. The combo of green herbs, garlic and eggs lends this dish a fresh and deep earthy flavour that is simply too good to be missed.

Preparation Time: 5 Minutes

Cooking Time: 12 Minutes

Servings: 2

Ingredients:

- 2 tablespoon Butter, preferably organic and pastured

- ¼ teaspoon Cayenne, grounded

- 1 tablespoon Coconut oil

- 4 Eggs, large and preferably organic

- 2 cloves of Garlic, chopped finely

- 1 teaspoon Thyme leaves, preferably fresh

- ½ cup Parsley, fresh and finely chopped

- ½ cup Cilantro, fresh and finely chopped

- ½ teaspoon Sea Salt

- ¼ teaspoon Cumin, grounded

Method of Preparation:

1) To begin with, take a non-stick pan and heat it over medium heat.

2) Next, stir in the butter and coconut oil into it and allow it to melt.

3) Once it is melted, add the chopped garlic and sauté it for two to three minutes or until it starts browning and becomes aromatic.

4) Now, spoon in the thyme and cook it again for further 20 seconds until it is lightly browned (Tip: Make sure not to burn the garlic.)

5) Then, add the parsley and cilantro to the pan and cook for about 2 to 3 minutes or until they are lightly crisp.

6) After that, crack the egg while making sure not to break the yolk.

7) Lower the heat and cover the pan and allow it to cook for about 5 to 6 minutes or until it is cooked and set.

8) Transfer it to the serving plate and enjoy it with your favourite side dishes like sausages.

Tip: If you prefer a runny one, cook the egg only for 3 to 4 minutes.

Nutritional Information

- ➢ Calories – 311 kcal
- ➢ Fat – 27.5gm
- ➢ Carbohydrates – 2.5gm
- ➢ Proteins – 12.8gm
- ➢ Fiber – 1gm

Eat Fat and Get Thin, Fit, and Healthier Than Ever Before!

Chorizo Breakfast Casserole

Have a big family to feed? Then this is a great recipe for an easy weekday breakfast the whole family will love. It is satisfyingly creamy cheese meal that is sure to become a family favorite because of its vibrant flavour!

Preparation Time: 20 Minutes

Cooking Time: 50 Minutes

Servings: 10

Ingredients:

- 16 oz. Chorizo, grounded
- 12 Medium Eggs, preferably organic
- 1 Onion, small and sliced finely
- 8 oz. Cheddar Cheese
- 1 teaspoon Onion Powder
- 1 Green Pepper, small and finely sliced
- 366 g or 1 ¼ to ½ cup Spinach
- ¾ cup Heavy Cream
- 1 teaspoon Garlic Powder
- Sea Salt and Pepper, to taste

Method of Preparation:

1) First, cook the spinach in the microwave.

2) Next, cook the grounded chorizo in a non-stick pan over medium-high heat and cook until it is browned.

3) Once it is done, transfer the browned chorizo into a large bowl.

4) After that, sauté the onion and pepper in the same skillet until the onion becomes translucent and softened.

5) Add the softened onion and pepper mixture along with the cooked spinach into the large bowl and combine them well.

6) Now, whisk together the eggs, the heavy cream and the spices in another medium-sized bowl until they are well combined.

7) Then, spoon in the heavy cream mixture into the large bowl and give it a good stir until everything is well

incorporated.

8) Finally, pour the mixture into the buttered casserole and bake it in the oven for 50 minutes at 350 degrees Fahrenheit.

Tip: It is also possible to add cherry tomatoes into the mixture.

Nutritional Information:

➢ Calories – 362 kcal

➢ Fat – 28gm

➢ Carbohydrates -7gm

➢ Proteins – 24gm

➢ Fiber – 2gm

Eat Fat and Get Thin, Fit, and Healthier Than Ever Before!

Crustless Two Cheese Quiche

Simple and straight forward, this light flavoured crustless quiche celebrate the sweet flavour of muenster and colby cheese and of the caramelized onion with a just set creamy filling!

Preparation Time: 10 Minutes

Cooking Time: 50 Minutes

Servings: 12

Ingredients:

- 3 cups Muenster Cheese, shredded
- 1 onion, large and chopped finely
- 2 cups Heavy Cream
- 3 cups Colby Cheese, shredded
- 2 tsp Thyme, dried
- 2 tablespoons Organic Butter, preferably pasteurised
- 1 teaspoon Sea Salt
- 12 Eggs, large and organic
- 1 teaspoon Black Pepper grounded

Method of Preparation:

1) To begin with, preheat the oven to 350 degrees Fahrenheit.

2) After that, heat a medium-sized skillet over medium-high heat and to this, add butter.

3) Once the butter has melted, stir in the onions and dried thyme into the pan and cook for 2 to 3 minutes or until the onion mixture is softened and transparent.

4) Next, apply butter on the two deep pie pans and then place 1 ½ cups of each of the cheeses into these pans.

5) Spread the onion mixture evenly over the cheese layer among the two pans.

6) Now, whisk the twelve eggs in a large bowl along with the heavy cream and ground pepper until they are well incorporated and frothy in texture.

7) Then, spoon half of the mixture into each of the pans and then with the help of a fork, lightly combine the cheese mixture and the egg mixture.

8) Finally, bake them for 23 to 25 minutes or until they are slightly golden colour in the middle and set.

9) Remove it from the oven and transfer it to the serving bowl.

10)   Serve it hot or cool it for some time and store it for later use.

Tip: This recipe is a freezer friendly recipe and can be kept for two weeks in the freezer.

Nutritional Information:

➢ Calories – 382 kcal
➢ Fat – 33gm
➢ Carbohydrates – 5gm
➢ Proteins – 16gm
➢ Fiber – 1gm

Eat Fat and Get Thin, Fit, and Healthier Than Ever Before!

Keto Breakfast Protein Smoothie

This is a delicious and a highly satiating smoothie recipe to throw together for breakfast when you don't have much time!On top, it is full of healthy fats and will maintain your energy till your lunch time!

Preparation Time: 5 Minutes

Cooking Time: 0 Minutes

Servings: 1

Ingredients:

- ½ cup Coconut Milk
- 1 tablespoon ground Chia Seeds
- ½ cup Water
- 1 tablespoon MCT Oil
- ¼ cup plain Whey Protein powder
- ½ teaspoon Cinnamon

Method of Preparation:

1) To begin with, place coconut milk, chia seeds, protein powder, cinnamon and MCT oil in the blender and blend until they become smooth and frothy. (Tip: you

can even add ice cubes.)

2) Transfer it to a serving glass and enjoy the delicious smoothie.

Tip: Instead of MCT oil, you can also use extra virgin coconut oil. But then, make sure to blend it well with the rest of the ingredients.

Nutritional Information:

- Calories – 467 kcal
- Fat – 40.3gm
- Carbohydrates – 4.7gm
- Proteins – 23.6gm
- Fiber – 3.5gm

Lunch and Dinner Recipes

Broccoli-Chicken Zucchini Boats

Serves: 2
Time: About 35 minutes

Zucchinis are fantastic substitutes for bread and make the perfect vehicle for all kinds of delicious ingredients. In this recipe, they hold chicken, tender broccoli, and melty cheese.

Ingredients:

2 hollowed-out, big zucchinis
6 ounces of shredded chicken
3 ounces of shredded Cheddar cheese
1 cup of broccoli
1 green onion stalk
2 tablespoons butter
2 tablespoons sour cream
Salt and pepper to taste

Directions:

1. Preheat your oven to 400-degrees.
2. Cut the zucchini in half, lengthwise, and hollow out with a spoon so you get a shell that's about 1-centimeter thick.
3. Pour 1 tablespoon of melted butter into the zucchini, sprinkle on salt and pepper, and put in the oven for 20

minutes.

4. In the meantime, shred the chicken and cut up your broccoli.

5. Mix with the sour cream and add salt and pepper.

6. When 20 minutes is up, fill the boats with the chicken-broccoli filling.

7. Sprinkle on the cheddar cheese and bake until the cheese has melted, about 10-15 minutes.

8. Top with chopped green onion and serve!

Nutritional Info:

Total calories: 476
Carbs: 5
Fat: 34
Protein: 30
Fiber: 3

Easiest Egg-Drop Soup

Serves: 1
Time: 5 minutes

This fast and tasty soup uses only a handful of ingredients, but packs a wallop, nutritionally-speaking. It's great for when you're feeling under the weather or want a simple breakfast or lunch.

Ingredients:

1 ½ cups chicken broth
½ cube chicken bouillon
2 big eggs
1 tablespoon butter
1 teaspoon chili garlic paste

Directions:

1. Get out a pan and heat it on medium-high.
2. Add chicken broth, butter, and bouillon cube.
3. When the broth is boiling, add the chili garlic paste and stir.
4. In a bowl, beat the eggs.
5. Pour in the broth and stir.
6. Let it set for a few seconds, and then serve!

Nutritional Info:

Total calories: 279
Carbs: 2.5
Fat: 23
Protein: 12
Fiber: 0

Portobello Pizzas

Serves: 4
Time: 10 minutes

Pizza is a very popular food, but it's usually not the healthiest option, and it's definitely not low-carb. However, by subbing out the usual bread crust with portobello mushroom caps and fresh tomato slices instead of sugar-filled tomato sauce, you get all the great flavors of pizza in a keto-friendly form!

Ingredients:

4 large portobello mushroom caps
20 slices of pepperoni
6 tablespoons olive oil
4 ounces of fresh mozzarella cheese
1 medium-sized tomato
¼ cup fresh, chopped basil
Salt and pepper to taste

Directions:

1. Scrape out the mushroom caps, so you just get a shell.
2. Brush the cap tops with olive oil and season with salt and pepper.
3. Broil for 4-5 minutes, then flip them over, and broil again.
4. In the meantime, slice the tomato into 12-16 slices.

5. Lay a few slices on each mushroom cap.
6. Add some basil leaves.
7. The last step is to add the pepperoni and a few cubes of mozzarella cheese.
8. Place under the broiler for another 2-4 minutes until the cheese begins to brown.
9. Cool before serving.

Nutritional Info:

Total calories: 321
Carbs: 2.8
Fat: 31
Protein: 8.5
Fiber: 1.2

Pork Chops w/ a Cumin Crust

Serves: 3
Time: Around 25-30 minutes

This recipe may look simple, but it has complex, rich flavors that will wow your taste buds. With just a few key spices, like cumin, coriander, and cardamom, ordinary pork chops are transformed into a meal you could serve for a dinner party.

Ingredients:

1 ½ pounds of pork chops
¼ cup golden flaxseed
2 stalks celery
1 orange pepper
½ white onion
¼ cup white wine
3 tablespoons coconut oil
2 teaspoons cumin
1 teaspoon cardamom
1 teaspoon coriander
Salt and pepper to taste

Directions:

1. Season the meat with salt and pepper.
2. Mix the flaxseed and spices together. These will form the crust.

3. Lay the chops in the crust mixture on both sides till well-coated.
4. Pour 3 tablespoons of coconut oil into a skillet and heat.
5. When the oil starts to smoke, put the pork chops in the skillet.
6. After 7 minutes, flip over, and cook for another 7 minutes on medium-low.
7. When the pork reaches 145-degrees, it's cooked through.
8. Wrap the chops in foil and rest on a pan.
9. Add the veggies to the pan with the meat juices.
10. Pour in the white wine and cook the veggies until they're soft.
11. Serve the pork chops with veggies.

Nutritional Info:

Total calories: 439
Carbs: 4.3
Fat: 23.7
Protein: 50.3
Fiber: 4.6

Oven-Baked Sweet + Sour Chicken

Serves: 4
Time: 65 minutes

This dish is usually full of sugar carbs, but thanks to the creative use of Erythritol, a naturally low-carb sweetener, you can have this lip-smacking meal on your ketogenic diet. Crushed pork rinds add an extra rich flavoring, too.

Ingredients:

5 pounds of boneless chicken breasts
1 cup crushed pork rinds
2 big, beaten eggs
½ cup almond flour
⅓ cup Parmesan cheese
2 tablespoons olive oil
1 tablespoon coconut oil
1 teaspoon salt
1 teaspoon black pepper

½ cup rice vinegar
½ cup Erythritol
4 tablespoons reduced-sugar ketchup
1 tablespoon soy sauce
1 teaspoon garlic powder

Directions:

1. Preheat your oven to 325-degrees.
2. Cut your chicken breasts into cubes.
3. Mix the crushed pork rinds with the almond flour, cheese, salt, and pepper.
4. In another bowl, beat the eggs.
5. Pour 1 tablespoon coconut oil and 1 tablespoon olive oil into a pan and heat.
6. Prepare the chicken cubes by dipping them first in the eggs, then the almond flour mixture.
7. Quickly brown the chicken in the pan before moving to a baking pan.
8. Mix the sauce (see second ingredient list) and pour over the chicken.
9. Bake in the oven for 60 minutes, stirring the chicken every 15 minutes.
10. Serve with mixed veggies or eat as is!

Nutritional Info (per 1.2 pound serving):

Total calories: 467
Carbs: 3.9
Fat: 32
Protein: 49
Fiber: 1.5

Walnut-Crusted Baked Salmon Fillets

Serves: 2
Time: 12 minutes

Salmon is one of the best foods you can eat on a keto diet. It's a fatty fish and cooks up in a flash. Using walnuts as a crust means even more great healthy fats, and using sugar-free maple syrup keeps it diet-friendly.

Ingredients:

2, 3-ounce salmon fillets
½ cup walnuts
2 tablespoons sugar-free maple syrup
1 tablespoon Dijon mustard
1 tablespoon olive oil
¼ teaspoon dill
Salt and pepper to taste

Directions:

1. Preheat your oven to 350 degrees.
2. Put the maple syrup, mustard, nuts, and seasonings into a food processor and run until it becomes a paste.
3. Heat the olive oil in a skillet until very hot.
4. Pat the salmon dry and lay it skin-side down to sear for 3 minutes.
5. As the fish sears, spread the walnut paste on the open face of the fillets.

6. After 3 minutes, move the pan to the oven and bake for 8 minutes.

7. Serve and enjoy!

Nutritional Info:

Total calories: 373
Carbs: 3
Fat: 43
Protein: 20
Fiber: 1

Nacho Chicken Casserole

Serves: 6
Time: About 30 minutes

If you love creamy and cheesy, this is the perfect casserole for you. It uses boneless, skinless chicken thighs, which are very affordable, and just one cup of those canned green chilies-and-tomatoes with some chili seasoning for the "nacho" part of the dish.

Ingredients:

1.75 pounds of boneless, skinless chicken thighs
4 ounces of cheddar cheese
4 ounces of cream cheese
1 packet of frozen cauliflower
1 medium-sized jalapeno pepper
1 cup green chilies and tomatoes
3 tablespoons Parmesan cheese
¼ cup sour cream
2 tablespoons olive oil
1 ½ teaspoons chili seasoning
Salt and pepper to taste

Directions:

1. Preheat your oven to 375-degrees.
2. Chop and season the chicken with salt and pepper.
3. Heat olive oil in a skillet before browning the chicken

over medium-high.

4. Add the sour cream, cream cheese, and ¾ of the cheddar into the skillet and stir until melted together.

5. Add in the chilies and green tomatoes.

6. Pour into a casserole dish.

7. Microwave the cauliflower until it is cooked through.

8. Blend with the rest of the cheese until smooth.

9. Cut the jalapeno.

10. Spread the cauliflower sauce over the casserole, then add the cut jalapeno on top in an even layer.

11. Bake for 15-20 minutes.

12. Serve hot!

Nutritional Info:

Total calories: 426
Carbs: 4.3
Fat: 32.2
Protein: 30.8
Fiber: 1.7

Crispy Baked Chicken Wings

Serves: 5
Time: 35 minutes (not counting overnight)

It's hard to get chicken wings really crispy if you don't have a deep-fryer. However, with just a few ingredients, this recipe produces amazingly crispy, no-carb wings from the oven!

Ingredients:

20 chicken wings and drumsticks
¼ cup butter
1 tablespoon salt
2 teaspoons baking powder
1 teaspoon baking soda

Directions:

1. Put all the wings in a plastic bag, along with the salt, baking soda, and baking powder.
2. Shake well.
3. Put the wings on a wire rack and put in the fridge overnight.
4. When you're ready to bake them, preheat the oven to 450-degrees.
5. Put the rack with the wings in the top middle position.
6. Bake for 20 minutes, then flip the wings over, and bake for another 15 minutes.

7. To serve, toss in the melted butter with some cilantro or other herbs.

Nutritional Info:

Total calories: 500
Carbs: 0
Fat: 38.8
Protein: 34
Fiber: 0

Chicken Parmesan

Serves: 4
Time: About 40 minutes

Chicken parm is an Italian classic. It's cheesy, crispy, and everything that good comfort food should be. To keep this recipe keto-friendly, use flaxseed meal instead of flour.

Ingredients:

3 chicken breasts
1 cup mozzarella cheese
Salt and pepper to taste

2.5 ounces of pork rinds
1 big egg
½ cup Parmesan cheese
¼ cup flaxseed meal
2 teaspoons paprika
1 ½ teaspoon chicken broth
1 teaspoon oregano
½ teaspoon salt
½ teaspoon pepper
½ teaspoon garlic
¼ teaspoon red pepper flakes

1 cup tomato sauce
¼ cup olive oil
Another ¼ cup olive oil

½ teaspoon oregano
½ teaspoon garlic
Salt and pepper to taste

Directions:

1. Put the flaxseed meal, parm cheese, spices, and pork rinds in a food processor and grind them into a coating.
2. Slice the chicken breasts in half, or pound into cutlets.
3. In a separate bowl, beat the egg with the chicken broth.
4. Mix all the ingredients in the third list in a saucepan and cook for 20 minutes.
5. In the meantime, dip the cutlets into the egg bowl, and then the coating.
6. Lay aside for now.
7. In another pan, heat 2 tablespoons of olive oil and fry the chicken. You may need more olive oil as it cooks.
8. Put the cooked chicken in a casserole dish, pour the sauce on top, and then add the mozzarella cheese on top.
9. Bake for just 10 minutes at 400-degrees until the cheese is melted.

Nutritional Info:

Total calories: 646
Carbs: 4
Fat: 46.8
Protein: 49.3
Fiber: 2.8

Korean Beef-Stuffed Peppers

Serves: 4
Time: 20-25 minutes
Stuffed bell peppers are a great alternative to hamburgers, especially when you fill the veggie with Korean barbeque. The beef is complimented with delicious ingredients like garlic, ginger, chili paste, and sugar-free apricot preserves for a spicy-sweet flavor.

Ingredients:

1 pound ground beef
8 big eggs
2 halved bell peppers
2 thinly-sliced spring onions
2 teaspoons minced ginger
2 teaspoons minced garlic
Salt and pepper to taste

⅓ cup sugar-free apricot preserves
1 ½ tablespoons rice wine vinegar
1 tablespoon chili paste
1 tablespoon soy sauce
1 tablespoons reduced-sugar ketchup

Directions:

1. Brown the beef on medium-high heat.
2. As it browns, season with salt, pepper, garlic, and ginger, and mix.

3. When meat is browned, push it aside, and add the sliced onions.

4. Let them fry for 1-2 minutes before removing the pan from the heat.

5. In another pan, mix all the ingredients in the second list and reduce, so it thickens.

6. Mix ½ of the sauce into the beef pan.

7. Stuff the pepper halves with the beef and cook at 350-degrees for 12-15 minutes.

8. While the peppers bake, fry the eggs.

9. When time is up, take out the peppers and brush the rest of the sauce on top.

10. Serve the peppers with two fried eggs per half.

Nutritional Info:

Total calories: 470
Carbs: 6.3
Fat: 35
Protein: 32.2
Fiber: 5.3

Easy Paprika Chicken

Serves: 4
Time: About 40 minutes

Paprika is an underused spice, in my opinion. In this recipe, it's the star, especially when you use Spanish smoked paprika. It adds a rustic, rich flavor that's complemented by bright lemon juice, sweet low-carb maple syrup, and garlic. For a side, steamed broccoli or sautéed spinach would be a good choice.

Ingredients:

4 boneless, skinless chicken breasts
3 tablespoons olive oil
2 tablespoons lemon juice
2 tablespoons Spanish smoked paprika
1 tablespoon low-carb maple syrup
2 teaspoons minced garlic
Salt and pepper to taste

Directions:

1. Preheat your oven to 350-degrees.
2. Cut the chicken into chunks and season with salt and pepper.
3. Mix the paprika, olive oil, garlic, and maple syrup together, making the sauce.
4. Spoon in ⅓ of the sauce into the bottom of a casserole dish

and put the chicken on top.

5. Pour the rest of the sauce evenly on top of the chicken.

6. Bake for 30-35 minutes.

7. Broil for another 4-5 minutes before serving.

Nutritional Info:

Total calories: 274
Carbs: 2
Fat: 13.6
Protein: 36.4
Fiber: 1.5

Shrimp + Mushroom Zoodles

Serves: 2
Time: 10-12 minutes

Using zucchini in place of regular pasta is my favorite diet hack. With this recipe, you toss the "zoodles" with white mushrooms, shrimp, a little marinara sauce, and seasonings like red pepper flakes and basil. It's the perfect summer supper.

Ingredients:

12 ounces of peeled shrimp
1 big zucchini
½ pound white mushrooms
½ cup marinara sauce
2 tablespoons olive oil
2 tablespoons butter
A dash of red pepper flakes
A sprinkle of Parmesan cheese
Basil
Oregano
Salt and pepper to taste

Directions:

1. Pour 2 tablespoons of oil into a skillet and heat.
2. Slice the mushrooms and fry them until they've soaked up most of the liquid.

3. Add in 2 tablespoons butter and keep cooking the mushrooms till they become golden.

4. Throw in the shrimp and cook for 4 minutes on each side.

5. While the shrimp cooks, use a spiralizer to make your zoodles.

6. When the shrimp is cooked through and pink, add the zoodles to the pan and mix. Cook for 2 minutes.

7. Pour in the marinara sauce and seasonings, and mix together.

8. Serve with Parmesan cheese!

Nutritional Info:

Total calories: 440
Carbs: 7.5
Fat: 28
Protein: 39
Fiber: 2.5

Chicken + Cauliflower Casserole w/ Vodka Sauce

Serves: 6
Time: 40 minutes

If you're in the mood for a rich dish that will warm you up on cold nights, this chicken casserole will hit the spot. It's got mushrooms, cauliflower, cheese, and calls for low-carb vodka sauce, which you can buy at the store.

Ingredients:

20 ounces of chicken breasts
2 cups riced cauliflower
2.5 ounces of mushrooms
1 ounce of pork rinds
1 cup chicken stock
1 cup shredded mozzarella cheese
½ cup low-carb vodka sauce
¼ cup heavy cream
¼ cup mayo
2 tablespoons Parmesan cheese
1 tablespoon olive oil
Oregano
Garlic powder
Salt and pepper to taste

Directions:

1. Preheat your oven to 375-degrees.

2. When the oven is ready, cook the chicken breasts for 20 minutes.

3. Heat the chicken broth until it's boiling.

3. Throw in the riced cauliflower and cook for 10-15 minutes, until all the liquid is gone.

4. When the chicken is cooked, shred with two forks.

5. Pour the heavy cream into the cauliflower and cook for another 5 minutes.

6. Slice the mushrooms and mix with the chicken with ¼ cup of mayo.

7. Add the cauliflower and stir.

8. Season.

9. Pour in the vodka sauce.

10. Transfer everything into a baking dish and press down to form an even layer.

11. Bake for 20 minutes.

12. Serve hot!

Nutritional Info:

Total calories: 300
Carbs: 2.5
Fat: 21
Protein: 29
Fiber: 0

Cucumber Sushi Rolls

Serves: 2
Time: 30 minutes

By using cucumber and forging rice, you can make refreshing, almost no-carb sushi rolls that are perfect for lunch! This recipe uses a good quality tuna steak, because you will be eating it raw, as well as creamy avocado, sriracha, green onion, and sesame seeds.

Ingredients:

2 cucumbers
½ pound tuna steak
½ avocado
2 tablespoons mayo
1 green onion stalk
2 teaspoons Sriracha
½ teaspoon sesame seeds
Directions:

1. Peel the cucumber and cut off the ends.
2. Choose a long, sharp knife, and run it under water, so it's wet.
3. Carefully cut along the outside of the cucumber; you should be able to just see the knife through the transparent fruit, so about 1/10 of an inch. You are basically cutting a "sheet" of cucumber, which you will roll.
4. When you've reached the seeds, you're done cutting.

5. Slice the raw tuna into thin squares, and the avocado into slices.

6. Mix the mayo and hot sauce together.

7. Spread out your cucumber roll and lay down the fish on one side. Top the fish with some avocado slices.

8. Roll tightly, beginning on the end with the fish.

9. When you've almost finished the roll, spread the spicy mayo on the cucumber and complete the roll, so the mayo sticks the roll together.

10. Cut the cucumber into ½-1 inch rounds.

11. Repeat with the second cucumber, so you get about 12 sushi pieces in total, which is enough for two people.

12. Garnish with chopped green onion and sesame seeds!

Nutritional Info:

Total calories: 322
Carbs: 2.5
Fat: 17
Protein: 36
Fiber: 3.9

Spicy Plum Tomato Soup

Serves: 6
Time: 1 hour, 20 minutes

This is no ordinary tomato soup. You roast the plum tomatoes in the oven, which gives them an unbelievably rich flavor, and then cook them with garlic and a sweet onion. You can adjust the spicier seasonings, or leave them out completely, if you really don't like too much heat. The whole thing is pureed, so the result is a hot, spicy, silky-smooth soup that would be perfect for cool days.

Ingredients:

3 pounds of plum tomatoes
1 quart of chicken broth
6 garlic cloves
1 sweet onion
½ cup basil
3 tablespoons olive oil
2 tablespoons butter
2 tablespoons tomato paste
1 tablespoon salt
1 tablespoon sriracha
1 teaspoon crushed red pepper
½ teaspoon thyme

½ teaspoon pepper
½ teaspoon paprika

Directions:

1. Divide up the plum tomatoes into thirds.
2. Wash and dry ⅓of the tomatoes and cut them in half, lengthwise.
3. Grease a baking sheet and arrange the cut tomatoes with the cut-side up.
4. Season with olive oil and salt.
5. Bake at 400-degrees for 40 minutes.
6. In the meantime, cut the onion and put the garlic through a garlic press.
7. Pour 1 tablespoon of olive oil in a large pot and cook the garlic and onion until translucent.
8. Cut the rest of the tomatoes into chunks (the fresh ones) and add them to the pot.
9. Pour in the broth and bring to a boil.
10. Toss in the basil leaves, along with butter and tomato paste.
11. Add the spices.
12. Bring to a boil on the stove.
13. When the tomatoes in the oven are roasted, put them in the pot and reduce the heat to a simmer.
14. After 40 minutes, pour into a large blender and process until creamy.
15. Pour into bowls and serve!

Nutritional Info:

Total calories: 164
Carbs: 9
Fat: 12
Protein: 3
Fiber: 2.7

Eat Fat and Get Thin, Fit, and Healthier Than Ever Before!

Clam Chowder

Serves: 4
Time: 45 minutes

Not only in this clam chowder low carb, it's gluten-free! By using cauliflower and xanthan gum as thickeners, this tasty chowder doesn't use any flour, and you can't tell the difference at all, taste-wise.

Ingredients:

½ head cauliflower
16-ounces of canned clams
2 ½ cups heavy cream
1 cup water
1 cup clam juice
3 strips bacon
4 garlic cloves
2 celery stalks
1 carrot
1 onion
2 tablespoons butter
1 teaspoon xanthan gum
1 teaspoon salt
1 teaspoon parsley
½ teaspoon thyme

½ teaspoon pepper
½ teaspoon celery salt

Directions:

1. Fill a pot with water to boil the cauliflower and heat.
2. When it's hot, chop up the cauliflower and put it in the pot to cook for 10 minutes until very soft.
3. In the meantime, cube the bacon and mince the onions and carrots.
4. Cut the celery into ¼-inch slices.
5. In a separate pot, cook the bacon until it's almost crispy, then add the onion, carrot, and celery.
6. Season with a little salt and cook until the onion is turning clear.
7. Add the garlic and butter.
8. Separate the canned clams and juice, saving the juice.
9. Drain the cauliflower and process in a blender until smooth.
10. Add the cauliflower, water, clam juice, and heavy cream into the bacon/veggies pot.
11. Reduce the heat and simmer for 20 minutes.
12. Season.
13. Add the xanthan gum and mix.
14. Add the clams and cook for just 5 minutes to avoid tough clams.
15.   Serve!

Eat Fat and Get Thin, Fit, and Healthier Than Ever Before!

Nutritional Info:

Total calories: 804
Carbs: 15
Fat: 66
Protein: 28
Fiber: 0

Eat Fat and Get Thin, Fit, and Healthier Than Ever Before!

Salmon Poke Bowl

Serves: 2
Time: 25 minutes

"Poke" is the term used for raw fish salad, and poke bowls are very popular in Hawaii. This poke bowl uses salmon, a great fatty fish, and seasonings like toasted sesame oil, fresh lemon juice, green onions, and coconut aminos, which is used in place of soy sauce. Instead of carb-heavy rice, you use *cauliflower* rice.

Ingredients:

½ pound sushi-grade, skinless, boneless salmon
2 chopped medium-sized green onions
2 tablespoons coconut aminos
1 tablespoon fresh lemon juice
1 tablespoon sesame seeds
1 tablespoon toasted sesame oil
1 teaspoon rice vinegar
1 teaspoon Sriracha

2 cups cauliflower rice
1 tablespoon rice vinegar
1 tablespoon coconut oil
¼ teaspoon salt

Directions:

1. Mix the coconut aminos, lemon juice, vinegar, salt, and toasted sesame oil together.
2. Cut the salmon into ½-1 inch pieces.
3. Put the fish in a bowl and pour in the marinade, along with the sesame seeds and green onions.
4. Add the sriracha and mix well.
5. Store in the fridge while you make the cauliflower rice.
6. Run the cauliflower through a food processor to get a grain-like texture that fills 2 cups.
7. Grease a pan with butter and heat.
8. When hot, put in the cauliflower rice and cook for 5-7 minutes, stirring so the rice doesn't stick and burn.
9. In a small bowl, mix salt and vinegar.
10. When the cauliflower is done, remove from heat and mix with the vinegar.
11. Serve the raw salmon on top, with your choice of toppings, including avocado slices, cucumber, daikon, and/or pickled ginger.

Nutritional Info:

Total calories: 400
Carbs: 8.5
Fat: 42.4
Protein: 30.3
Fiber: 8.8

Steak w/ Mustard Sauce

Serves: 2
Time: 30-40 minutes

This recipe serves two, so it would be a great dinner for a summer date night. You pan-sear (or oven-cook) two boneless strip steaks, and dress it with an awesome creamy mustard + peppercorn sauce that you'll want to lick off the plate.

Ingredients:

2 medium-sized boneless strip steaks
1 tablespoon lard
Salt and pepper to taste

1 tablespoon Dijon mustard
1 tablespoon lard
1 tablespoon whole black peppercorns
¼ cup coconut milk
¼ cup chicken stock
½ teaspoon onion powder
Salt to taste

Directions:

1. Season the steaks with salt and pepper.
2. Heat the lard in a cast-iron skillet and lay down the steaks.

3. Cook for about 3 minutes on each side, or until nice and brown, depending on the thickness.

4. When cooked, move to a wire rack and cover them loosely with foil.

5. Rest for 10 minutes.

6. In the meantime, make the sauce with the ingredients listed in the second ingredient list.

7. Add the ghee to the steak pan to melt.

8. With a rolling pin, crush the peppercorns.

9. Add to the pan and cook for 2-3 minutes, until they become fragrant.

10. Toss in the onion powder, broth, cream, and mustard.

11. Reduce the heat to medium, and bring to a boil.

12. Let the liquid reduce by half, and then cook for 3-5 minutes until the sauce is creamy.

13. Serve the steak with the sauce and enjoy!

Nutritional Info:

Total calories: 600
Carbs: 3.3
Fat: 65.2
Protein: 39.5
Fiber: 1.4

Spaghetti Squash w/ Beef Meatballs

Serves: 10
Time: 1 hour, 25 minutes

Spaghetti with meatballs is pretty much off-limits if you're on a keto diet. However, by replacing pasta noodles with spaghetti squash, you get a nutritious substitute that tastes awesome! The beef meatballs are also delicious, and each person gets three.

Ingredients:

48 ounces of ground beef
1 onion
1 green pepper
8 ounces shredded cheddar cheese
3 egg
3 tablespoon coconut flour
3 tablespoon minced garlic
Salt and pepper

1 cooked and shredded spaghetti squash
24 ounces marinara sauce
10 teaspoons Parmesan cheese

Directions:

1. To cook the squash, begin by cutting the fruit in half and scraping out the inside.

2. Put face down on a glass baking dish and add enough water to cover the line where the squash has been cut.
3. Cook for 45 minutes at 375-degrees.
4. Cut up the onions and pepper.
5. Mix the pepper/onions, the beef, coconut flour, egg, cheese, garlic, salt, and pepper.
6. Form 30 meatballs and put on a foil-lined pan.
7. Bake for 25 minutes in the oven with the squash.
8. When the meat is 165-degrees, it's ready.
9. When the squash is done, use a fork to scrape out "noodles" and plate.
10. Add the meatballs and mix with tomato sauce.
11. Top with cheese!

Nutritional Info:

Total calories: 306
Carbs: 13
Fat: 21
Protein: 45
Fiber: 3

Slow-Cooker BBQ Chicken

Serves: 4
Time: 6 hours, 45 minutes

Slow cookers are a great way to make fork-tender BBQ chicken. You can pile the chicken on a salad instead of in a sandwich, to keep things keto-friendly.

Ingredients:

6 boneless, skinless chicken thighs
⅓ cup salted butter
¼ cup red wine vinegar
¼ cup Erythritol
¼ cup organic tomato paste
¼ cup chicken stock
2 tablespoons spicy brown mustard
2 tablespoons yellow mustard
1 tablespoon soy sauce
1 tablespoon liquid smoke
2 teaspoons chili powder
1 teaspoon cayenne pepper
1 teaspoon cumin
1 teaspoon Red Boat fish sauce

Directions:

1. Add the butter, chicken stock, vinegar, tomato paste, mustards, liquid smoke, soy sauce, fish sauce, and

seasonings into a bowl.

2. Add the Erythritol sweetener and mix well.

3. Taste and adjust to your liking. More vinegar makes the sauce tangier, while more sweetener makes it sweeter.

4. Put the chicken thighs in the slow cooker and pour over the BBQ sauce.

5. Cook for 2 hours.

6. Open the lid and push down on the chicken, so it's beneath the juices.

7. Add the butter and swirl it around, so it gets on the chicken.

8. Cook for another 3-4 hours.

9. Shred the chicken.

10. With the lid on, keep cooking on high for another 45 minutes to reduce the sauce.

11. Mix one last time before serving!

Nutritional Info:

Total calories: 510
Carbs: 2.3
Fat: 30
Protein: 51.5
Fiber: 0

Chicken Cordon Bleu Casserole

Serves: 10
Time: 40-45 minutes

Chicken cordon bleu just *sounds* intimidating. It's in the name of the largest cooking school in the world, after all. However, making the French classic in casserole form is shockingly easy, and just as delicious.

Ingredients:

53 ounces of chicken breasts, tenders, or thighs
300 grams of ham steak
11 ounces of Jarlsberg swiss cheese
1 cup of heavy whipping cream
1 cup cream cheese
Garlic powder
Salt and pepper to taste

Directions:

1. Cut the chicken into 1-inch cubes and lay on the bottom of a pan.
2. Season the chicken.
3. Cut the ham into ½-inch cubes and put on top of the chicken.
4. Shred the cheese over the meat.
5. Put the cream cheese in the microwave and then stir in the cream, so it makes a sauce.

6. Pour into the pan and mix.

7. Bake in a 350-degree oven for 40 minutes.

8. Serve hot!

Nutritional Info:

Total calories: 486
Carbs: 4
Fat: 30
Protein: 38
Fiber: 0

Sunflower-Butter Pork Kabobs

Serves: 4
Time: 1 hour, 15 minutes

Sunflower butter is made from sunflower seeds, and has that same nutty-sweet, summery flavor. It's less intense than peanut butter, so the other flavors in the pork like the hot sauce, garlic, and crushed red pepper really come through.

Ingredients:

1 pound pork
1 medium-sized green bell pepper
3 tablespoons sunflower butter
1 tablespoon minced garlic
1 tablespoon soy sauce
1 tablespoon water
2 teaspoons hot sauce (like Sriracha)
½ teaspoon crushed red pepper

Directions:

1. Mix everything but the pork in a food processor until smooth.
2. Cut the pork into bite-sized pieces and mix in a bowl with the marinade.
3. Let the pork marinate for at least 1 hour.
4. Chop the green pepper into skewer-ready pieces.

5. Skewer the meat and pepper alternately on metal skewers.

6. Broil for five minutes per side on high until the meat is 145-degrees.

7. Serve and enjoy!

Nutritional Info (1 kabob):

Total calories: 200
Carbs: 5
Fat: 8
Protein: 24
Fiber: 2

Tequila-Marinated Chicken

Serves: 6
Time: 3 hours, 38 minutes

For an unforgettable summer meal, how about chicken with the flavors of a tequila shot? We're talkin' lime juice, salt, and of course, tequila. There's also a fantastic sauce that goes along with it, which includes dill, hot sauce, cream, and an array of spices. Those flavors bake together in an oven, covered with cheese.

Ingredients:

6 chicken breasts
1 cup water
50 mL tequila
¼ cup soy sauce
2 tablespoons lime juice
½ teaspoon liquid smoke
½ teaspoon garlic powder
½ teaspoon salt

6 ounces of shredded cheddar cheese
¼ cup salsa
¼ cup sour cream
¼ cup mayonnaise
1 tablespoon heavy cream
¼ teaspoon hot sauce
¼ teaspoon dried parsley

¼ teaspoon salt
¼ teaspoon paprika
¼ teaspoon dried parsley
¼ teaspoon dill
¼ teaspoon ground cumin
¼ teaspoon black pepper
¼ teaspoon cayenne pepper

Directions:

1. Mix all the ingredients from the first list in a large Zip-loc bag.
2. Let the chicken marinade for 2-3 hours in the fridge.
3. When time is up, lay the chicken on a broiler pan and broil for 20 minutes, 10 minutes on each side.
4. When the chicken is 165-degrees, transfer to a casserole dish.
5. Mix all the ingredients in the second list (except the cheese) and pour over the chicken.
6. Top with the shredded cheese and broil for another 3 minutes.

Nutritional Info:

Total calories: 445
Carbs: 2
Fat: 22
Protein: 60
Fiber: 0

Nutty Almond Stromboli

What's not to love about this golden crusted low carb Stromboli? Loaded with cheese and nut flours, this main course meal is a total crowd pleaser!

Preparation Time: 20 Minutes

Cooking Time: 30 Minutes

Servings: 5

Ingredients:

- 4 tablespoon Almond Flour
- 1 ¼ cup Mozzarella cheese, shredded
- 1 Egg, preferably large and organic
- 3 tablespoon Coconut Flour
- 1/8 teaspoon Garlic powder
- 4 tablespoon Butter, melted
- 1 teaspoon Red Pepper flakes
- ¼ teaspoon Fennel powder

For the Filling:

- 14 slices of Pepperoni
- ½ cup Mozzarella Cheese, shredded

Method of Preparation:

1) To start with, preheat the oven to 400 degrees Fahrenheit.

2) After that, place the butter in a small bowl and melt it in the microwave.

3) Next, combine the shredded mozzarella cheese with the red pepper flakes, fennel powder and garlic powder in a large bowl and melt it in the microwave for about two minutes at lower power.

4) Now, combine almond flour, egg, melted butter and coconut flour until they are mixed well .

5) Then, stir together the almond flour mixture into the melted cheese mixture and combine until they are well incorporated. Microwave the mixture for further 20 to 30 seconds. (Microwaving the mixture again helps to blend them better.)

6) Microwave the dough again for another 10 to 20 seconds.

7) To roll the dough, place parchment paper on the working station and then roll out the dough into a rectangle shape.

8) Now, slice the long sides straight with the help of a pizza cutter.

9) After that, cut through the strips on each side evenly while leaving space in the centre for the filling.

10) Finally, place the cheese and the slices of pepperoni in the middle and place the strips over it.

11) Then, fold up the dough so as to get the Stromboli shape.

12) Finally, bake it for 14 to 20 minutes at 400 degrees Fahrenheit until it becomes golden brown in colour.

Tip: For all the cheeses that come with a higher fat content, you may need to add more of coconut flour to make it more stable.

Eat Fat and Get Thin, Fit, and Healthier Than Ever Before!

Nutritional Information:

- ➤ Calories – 1184 kcal
- ➤ Fat – 102gm
- ➤ Carbohydrates – 5gm
- ➤ Proteins – 13gm
- ➤ Fiber – 2gm

Breadless BLT Sandwich

This fare makes for a satisfyingly breadless sandwich that is sure to please your taste buds. High on flavour and heat with spicy sauce and seasonings, this dish is sure to warm your heart.

Preparation Time: 10 Minutes

Cooking Time: 30 Minutes

Servings: 2

- Ingredients:
- 3 Eggs, preferably organic and large
- ½ teaspoon Garlic Powder
- 3 oz. Cream Cheese
- ¼ teaspoon Sea Salt
- 1/8 teaspoon Cream of Tartar

<u>To make the filling:</u>

- 1 tablespoon Mayonnaise
- 3 oz. Chicken
- 2 Grape Tomatoes, halved
- 1 teaspoon Sriracha
- 2 Bacon slices
- ¼ of 1 Avocado, medium sized and mashed slightly

- 2 Pepper Jack Cheese slices

Method of Preparation:

1) First, preheat the oven to 300 degrees Fahrenheit.

2) After that, take two medium sized bowls. Place egg white and egg yolk into these two bowls respectively.

3) Next, stir in the salt and cream of tartar into the egg whites and whisk them with the help of an egg beater until you get foamy and soft peaks.

4) Now, spoon in the cream of cheese into the egg yolk and combine until they are well combined.

5) Then, fold the egg white mixture into the cream cheese mixture gradually until they are well incorporated.

6) Once it is mixed, ladle about a quarter of a cup of the mixture into a baking sheet which is lined with parchment paper and then press them slightly so as to get a square shape. Add garlic powder on the top and then bake it for 22 to 23 minutes.

7) In the meantime, heat a non-stick pan over medium-high heat and then add oil once it is hot.

8) To this add the chicken and bacon along with a bit of salt and pepper and cook until is cooked.

9) Take the keto bread out of the oven and allow it to cool.

10) Spread the Sriracha and the mayonnaise together into one side of the keto bread.

11) Finally, place the chicken mixture on top of the mayonnaise. Top it with the cheese slices, tomato and mashed avocado.

12) Cover it with the second keto bread and transfer it to a serving plate.

13) Enjoy it hot along with your choice of seasoning.

Tip: Make sure to whip the egg white carefully and slowly since it affects the texture of the bread much.

Nutritional Information:

Eat Fat and Get Thin, Fit, and Healthier Than Ever Before!

- ➤ Calories – 361 kcal
- ➤ Fat – 28.3gm
- ➤ Carbohydrates – 2g
- ➤ Proteins – 22gm

Baked Squash and Beef Lasagna

Want a comfort food without guilt? Then, this plate of hot baked goodness with the mild tasting squash and beef is sure to provide you a healthy and joyous eating.

Preparation Time: 10 Minutes

Cooking Time: 80 Minutes

Servings: 12

Ingredients:

- 2 large Spaghetti Squash, cooked
- 30 Slices of Mozzarella Cheese
- 3 Lbs Beef, grounded
- 40 Oz. Marinara sauce
- 32 Oz Ricotta Cheese, whole milk

Method of Preparation:

1) To start with, preheat the oven to 375-degree Fahrenheit.

2) Next, divide the squash into two pieces carefully.

3) After that, place the squash with the face down in a large sized glass dish and fill it with water until the

meat portion is covered.

4) Now, bake it in the oven for about 40 to 45 minutes or until the insides can be taken easily with a fork.

5) In the meantime, heat a skillet with a little bit of oil over medium-high heat.

6) To this, add the beef and cook until it is brown in colour.

7) Then, spoon in the marinara sauce and combine them well for about 3 to 5 minutes. Remove it from the heat and keep it aside.

8) At this point, scrape the insides of the squash to get the spaghetti for this recipe.

9) Next, add the squash into the bottom of the buttered large sized pan.

10) Top it with meat sauce, and then with the both kinds of cheese with the mozzarella cheese coming first and ricotta second.

11) Continue the process until all the ingredients are being used up.

12) Finally, bake it in the oven for about 30 to 35 minutes or until it becomes golden yellow in colour and the liquid cheese starts bubbling. Allow it to cool for few minutes and then serve it.

Tip: You will know the spaghetti is properly cooked when the insides break apart quickly.

Nutritional Information:
- ➢ Calories – 711 kcal
- ➢ Fat – 59g
- ➢ Carbohydrates – 15g
- ➢ Proteins – 43g
- ➢ Fiber – 2g

Eat Fat and Get Thin, Fit, and Healthier Than Ever Before!

Cauliflower Ham Casserole

If you are looking for something that looks like it might be decadent, but is really low carb and won't cause a problem as you are trying to slim down, this dish will be perfect!

Preparation Time: 20 Minutes

Cooking Time: 70 Minutes

Servings: 6

Ingredients:

- large head of 1 Cauliflower, cut into small florets, discarding leaf and core
- ¾ cup Cheddar Cheese, grated
- 4 oz. Cream Cheese, preferably reduced fat and softened
- ½ teaspoon Sea Salt
- 2 tablespoon Parmesan cheese, grated finely
- 2 cups lean Ham, diced
- ¼ cup Green Onions, sliced thinly
- ¾ cup Greek yoghurt
- Black Pepper, freshly grounded, to taste

Method of Preparation:

1) To start with, preheat the oven to 350 degrees Fahrenheit.

2) Then, take a deep bottomed pan and fill it with water half-way.

3) To this, add salt and bring the water to a boil.

4) Once it starts boiling, add the cauliflower florets and cook until it is cooked. (Make sure not over to cook it, since it will be cooked while it is being baked.

5) In the meantime, place the cream cheese in a medium-sized bowl and microwave it for one to two minutes or until it is softened.

6) Next, combine the softened cream cheese, green onion, yoghurt and parmesan and mix them well. Set it aside.

7) Remove the pot from the heat and then drain the water from it. Drain the cauliflower at least 3 to 5 minutes in a colander.

8) Now, with the help of a potato masher, mash the cooked cauliflower in the pan.

9) Once it is properly mashed, spoon in the cream cheese sauce and stir it well until the sauce coats the mashed cauliflower well.

10) Next, add the diced ham to it and mix and then season it with the freshly grounded black pepper.

11) Finally, pour the cauliflower mixture into a baking sheet lined with butter and spread it evenly. Top it with the grated cheese throughout.

12) Then, bake it for 28 to 34 minutes or until it becomes golden yellow in colour. At this point, the cheese would be melted and bubbling.

13) Allow it to sit for 10 to 15 minutes and then enjoy the highly delectable dish.

Tip: Instead of yoghurt, you can also use sour cream.

Nutritional Information:

- ➢ Calories – 160 kcal
- ➢ Fat – 8g
- ➢ Carbohydrates – 4g
- ➢ Proteins – 15g
- ➢ Fiber – 1gm

Spectacular Seafood and Bacon

The ingredients in this dish are few and simple as the seafood in it gives it most of its delicious flavour. Simple ingredients in just the right amount makes this fare easy to make and scrumptious to eat.

Preparation Time: 5 Minutes

Cooking Time: 15 Minutes

Servings: 4

Ingredients:

- 4 slices Bacon, organic and uncured, sliced into small pieces
- 4 oz Shrimp, raw and shelled
- 1 cup Mushrooms, sliced
- ½ cup heavy Whipping Cream (optional)
- 4 oz Salmon, smoked and cut into strips
- 1 pinch of Celtic Sea Salt
- Black pepper, freshly grounded

Method of Preparation:

- First, heat a non-stick skillet over medium heat.

- Then, add the bacon to the pan and cook until is done. (Tip :Do not make it crisp.)

- Now, stir in the mushroom and cook for about another 3 to 5 minutes.

- Next, spoon in the smoked salmon and saute it for about 2 to 4 minutes.

- After that, add the shrimp and raise the heat to high.

- Then, sauté it for further 3 to 4 minutes until it becomes transparent. To this, stir in the cream and salt.

- Finally, lower the heat and cook for another one minute.

- Serve it hot along with zucchini noodles (optional).

Tip: Instead of whipping cream, you can use coconut milk also.

Nutritional Information:

- ➤ Calories – 340 kcal
- ➤ Fat – 29g
- ➤ Carbohydrates – 3.5g
- ➤ Proteins – 17g
- ➤ Fiber – 1gm

Eat Fat and Get Thin, Fit, and Healthier Than Ever Before!

Amazing Avocado Recipes

Smoked Salmon Frittata with Avocado

Preparation time: 1 5 minutes
Cooking time: 10 minutes
Serves: 4

Ingredients:

- 1 tablespoon of grass fed ghee
- 6 free range eggs, beaten
- 1 large fillet of smoked salmon, flaked
- Salt and black pepper, to taste
- 1 teaspoon mixed Italian herbs
- 1 large tomato, diced
- 1 medium red onion, diced
- 1 stem of green onion, chopped

Directions:

- ➢ In a skillet, apply medium-low heat and add the ghee. Swirl to coat the skillet evenly with ghee and sauté the onions and tomatoes until soft and tender.
- ➢ Stir in the flaked salmon and Italian herbs, cook for 3 minutes and transfer to plate.
- ➢ Season the egg mixture with salt and pepper and pour into the skillet. Swirl to coat evenly the bottom of the skillet add the salmon-vegetable mixture.
- ➢ Reduce to the low heat, cover the skillet and cook until the

bottom is lightly golden and the edges starts to pull away.
➤ Slide unto a serving plate, cut into four wedges and top with green onions serving.

Spinach Omelet and Avocado

Preparation Time: 10 minutes
Serves: 1

Ingredients:

- 2 eggs (best if you can purchase them from a local farmer's market)
- 2 Avocados
- Handful of organic spinach
- Big pinch of parsley

Directions:

1. Mix the yolks and egg whites in a bowl (or discard the yolks if you prefer).
2. Pour eggs into a frying pan heated to medium-low. Heat until eggs are no longer runny, at least 3 minutes.
3. Top with spinach leaves and parsley.
4. Slice both avocados in half, garnish, and serve.

Eat Fat and Get Thin, Fit, and Healthier Than Ever Before!

Taco-Spiced Turkey Burrito

Preparation time: 10 minutes
Cooking time: 15 minutes
Serves: 4

Ingredients:

- 1 pound free range ground turkey
- 1 tablespoon of taco seasoning
- 1 teaspoon poultry seasoning
- Salt and black pepper, to taste
- 1 tablespoons grass fed ghee
- 4 gluten-free flour tortillas
- 1 red sweet pepper, minced
- 1 medium white onion, minced
- 1 stem green onions, chopped
- 2 tablespoons of salsa
- 1 ripe tomato, sliced
- 1 ripe avocado, sliced

Directions:

- ➤ Add the ground turkey, taco and poultry seasoning in a bowl. Season to taste with salt and pepper and mix until well combined.
- ➤ Add the ghee in a medium skillet and apply medium-high heat. Cook the ground turkey until lightly brown and cooked through. Remove from skillet and add the sweet pepper, white onion and green onions in the same skillet, sauté for about 5 minutes. Remove from pan, transfer to

136

the bowl with the ground turkey and mix until well combined.

➢ In the same pan, heat the tortillas for 1 minute on each side and place it on a flat work surface.

➢ Divide the meat mixture, salsa, tomato and avocado on each tortilla and roll up to form into burritos. Slice into halves, transfer to a serving plate and serve immediately.

Mexican Benedict Chipotle Sauce

Preparation time: 10 minutes
Cooking time: 5 minutes
Serves: 4

Ingredients:

- 2 chipotle peppers, seeded and diced
- 3 free range organic egg yolks
- ½ tablespoon of lime juice
- ½ cup of ghee
- 4 poached free range eggs
- 1 tablespoon of olive oil
- 4 cups loosely packed baby spinach
- Salt and ground black pepper, to taste

For Serving:
- ➤ 1 avocado, sliced
- ➤ 2 tablespoons minced fresh cilantro

Directions:

- Add the chipotle, egg yolks and lime juice in a blender and blend until smooth and well incorporated. Pulse again while gradually adding the ghee until a thick and smooth consistency is achieved.
- In a skillet, apply medium-high heat and add the oil. Add the spinach and cook for 3 minutes or until wilted. Season to taste with salt and pepper.
- Portion the spinach into 4 serving plates, top with poached

egg and drizzle with sauce on top.
- Serve warm with avocado slices and cilantro.

Turkey Breast Avocado Sandwich

Preparation time: 15 minutes
Cooking time: 15 minutes
Serves: 4

Ingredients:

- ➤ 1 free range organic turkey breast half, thinly sliced
- ➤ Salt and pepper, to taste
- ➤ 1 teaspoon of poultry seasoning
- ➤ 1 tablespoon of ghee
- ➤ 8 slices of gluten-free sandwich bread
- ➤ 2 tablespoons of green chili sauce

Toppings:
- ➤ Avocado slices
- ➤ Tomato slices
- ➤ Lettuce leaves
- ➤ Fried egg (optional)

DIRECTIONS:

- Rub the meat with salt, pepper and poultry seasoning on both sides. Add the ghee in a skillet over medium-high heat and fry the turkey breast for 4 minutes on each side. Remove from skillet and let it rest for 10 minutes before slicing.
- Spread the chili sauce on one side of four slices of bread, place the pan-fried turkey and add the toppings.
- Cut the sandwich across the diagonal, add fried egg (optional) transfer to a serving platter and serve.

Eat Fat and Get Thin, Fit, and Healthier Than Ever Before!

Salmon, Avocado and Cucumber Green Salad

Preparation time: 10 minutes
Cooking time: 10 minutes
Serves: 2

Ingredients:

- 1 fillet wild Atlantic salmon, skinless
- ¼ teaspoon garlic powder
- ¼ teaspoon Italian seasoning
- Salt and black pepper, to taste
- 1 lime, juiced
- 2 teaspoons grass fed ghee
- 2 cups loosely packed fresh kale, cut into chiffonade
- 1 ripe avocado, cubed
- 1 small cucumber, sliced into rounds
- 2 tablespoons minced parsley

For the Dressing:
- 2 tablespoons of olive oil
- 1 lime, juiced
- Salt and pepper
- 1 tablespoon minced dill

Directions:

1. Season the salmon with salt, pepper, garlic powder and Italian seasoning and drizzle with lime juice on both sides.
2. Add the ghee in a skillet over medium-high heat and fry the salmon for about 3 minutes on each side. Remove

from skillet, let it rest for 5 minutes on a plate and cut into cubes.

3. Whisk all dressing ingredients in a large bowl, add in the rest of the ingredients and gently toss to evenly coat the salad ingredients with dressing.

4. Divide into four serving bowls, top with salmon and serve immediately.

Spice-Rubbed Chicken with Avocado Salsa

Preparation time: 15 minutes
Cooking time: 15 minutes
Serves: 4

Ingredients:

- ➢ 4 free range organic chicken breasts halves (boneless and skinless)
- ➢ 1 tablespoon of olive oil

For the Spice rub:
- ½ teaspoon ground cumin
- 1 teaspoon of chili powder
- 1 teaspoon of smoked paprika
- ½ teaspoon of garlic powder
- Salt and coarsely ground pepper, to taste

For the Avocado Salsa:
- 1 cup of diced red tomato
- 1 cup avocado, pitted and diced
- ½ cup diced cucumber
- ¼ cup diced onion
- ¼ cup minced cilantro
- 2 tablespoons lime juice
- Salt and pepper

Directions:

1. Combine together all spice rub ingredients in a large bowl

and add the chicken. Rub the spice mixture evenly on all sides and set aside.

2. Mix together all ingredients for the avocado salsa in a separate bowl, season to taste with salt and pepper and toss to combine. Cover bowl and chill before serving.

3. In a medium skillet, apply medium-high heat and add the oil. Add and cook the chicken for 10 to 12 minutes while stirring occasionally, or until the meat is thoroughly cooked.

4. Portion the chicken on individual serving plates and serve with avocado salsa on top.

Fresh Snapper Ceviche

Preparation time: 15 minutes
Cooking time: 20 minutes
Serves: 2

Ingredients:

- Approximately 750g of fresh snapper, ensure all bones are removed and cut the meat into small cubes between 1 and 1.5 cm each
- Juice from three fresh, medium sized limes
- 1.5 cups of coconut water
- 2 tablespoons of coriander leaves, chopped
- 2 tablespoons of mint leaves, chopped
- 4 spring onions, sliced fine
- 1 small red chili, sliced fine
- Pinch of ground course sea salt

SALSA INGREDIENTS (if using as a dip)
- 1 ripe avocado, dice the flesh of the avocado into cubes of 1-2 cm each
- 1 red capsicum, diced
- 2 tablespoons chopped coriander
- Juice from half a lime (lime zest to taste)

Directions:

1. Mix herbs, chili, lime juice, coconut water, and spring onions, in small bowl.
2. Add fish to mix and ensure all cubes are thoroughly coated.
3. Cover and refrigerate for 3-5 hours.

4. Garnish with additional coriander and mint to taste. Serve on it's own or as a dip with your favorite vegetables, or shrimp if you want additional protein.

Greek Meatballs with Avocado Tzatziki Sauce

Preparation time: 15 minutes
Cooking time: 25 minutes
Serves: 4

Ingredients:

For the Meatballs:
- 1 pound ground grass-fed beef
- 1 small red onion, minced
- 1 ½ teaspoons minced garlic
- 1 organic lemon, zested
- 1 teaspoon of dried oregano
- ½ teaspoon cumin powder
- ½ teaspoon of coriander powder
- Pink Himalayan salt and pepper, to taste

For the Sauce:
- 1 avocado, diced
- 1 cucumber, diced
- 1 teaspoon minced garlic
- 1 tablespoon minced red onion
- 1 lemon, juiced
- 2 teaspoons minced dill
- Salt and black pepper, to taste

Directions:
1. Preheat an oven to a temperature of 350°F. Lightly grease

a baking pan with oil and set aside.
2. Combine all meatball ingredients until well combined and from into 2-inch balls. Transfer on the prepared baking pan and bake for 25 minutes, or until lightly browned and cooked through.
3. While cooking the meatballs, add all sauce ingredients in a food processor and pulse until smooth. Transfer to a bowl and set aside.
4. When the meatballs are done. Transfer into a serving platter and pour Tzatziki sauce over the meatballs. Serve immediately.

Baked Salmon with Avocado Salsa

Preparation time: 10 minutes
Cooking time: 15 minutes
Serves: 4 to 6

Ingredients:

- 3 fillets of wild Atlantic salmon
- 1 tablespoon of onion powder
- 1 teaspoon of Spanish paprika
- 1 teaspoon of ground cumin
- Salt and crushed black pepper, to taste
- 2 tablespoons of ghee or olive oil

For the Salsa:

- 2 ripe avocados, pitted and diced
- ½ cup of minced onions
- 2 jalapeno peppers, seeded and minced
- 3 organic limes, juiced
- 2 tablespoons of extra virgin olive oil
- 2 tablespoons of minced fresh cilantro leaves
- Salt and crushed black pepper, to taste

Directions:

1. Combine all salsa ingredients in a large bowl and set aside. Cover the bowl with plastic wrap and chill before using.
2. Preheat the oven to a temperature of 400°F. Lightly grease a baking pan with oil and set aside.
3. Combine all spices in a small bowl and rub evenly on both

sides of the salmon. Place the salmon on the prepared baking pan and drizzle with clarified butter on top of the salmon. Bake it in the oven for 15 minutes or until the fish flakes easily with a fork and cooked through. Remove from the oven and transfer on a serving plate.

4. Serve baked salmon warm with avocado salsa.

Vegan Tofu Tacos

Preparation time: 15 minutes
Cooking time: 15 minutes
Serves: 2 to 4

Ingredients:

- 1 cup of cooked black beans
- 8 ounces of firm tofu
- Half a medium sized red onion, diced
- 1 cup fresh cilantro, chopped
- 1 or 2 sliced avocados
- 0.25 cup of pomegranate seeds
- Half a cup of salsa
- Corn tortillas

SEASONING FOR TOFU:
- Half a teaspoon of chili powder
- 1 teaspoon of cumin
- 1 teaspoon of garlic powder
- Pinch of ground course sea salt
- 1 tablespoon of salsa
- 1 tablespoon of water

Directions:

1. Wrap tofu in a clean, absorbent towel and place something heavy on top, such as a cast iron skillet, while prepping toppings.
2. Cook black beans according to instructions on package, add a pinch each of salt, chili powder, cumin, and garlic

powder, then set aside.
3. Add the tofu seasoning and salsa to a bowl and top with just enough water to make a sauce that can be poured, then set aside.
4. Heat a pan over medium heat and add 1-2 tablespoons of oil and chopped tofu. Cook for 5 minutes, stirring frequently, then add seasoning. Cook for another 8 minutes, still stirring frequently.
5. Warm the tortillas and fill them with all of the ingredients, then serve and enjoy!

Sliced Chicken Burrito

Preparation time: 10 minutes
Cooking time: 15 minutes
Serves: 4

Ingredients:

- 1 pound of sliced chicken breasts
- 1 tablespoon of taco seasoning
- 1 teaspoon poultry seasoning
- Salt and black pepper, to taste
- 1 tablespoons grass fed ghee
- 4 gluten-free flour tortillas
- 1 red sweet pepper, minced
- 1 medium white onion, minced
- 1 stem green onions, chopped
- 2 tablespoons of salsa
- 1 ripe tomato, sliced
- 1 ripe avocado, sliced

Directions:

- Add the sliced chicken, taco and poultry seasoning in a bowl. Season to taste with salt and pepper and mix until well combined.
- Add the ghee in a medium skillet and apply medium-high heat. Cook the sliced chicken until until white and cooked through. Remove from skillet and add the sweet pepper, white onion and green onions in the same skillet, sauté for about 5 minutes. Remove from pan, transfer to the bowl with the sliced chicken and mix until well combined.

- In the same pan, heat the tortillas for 1 minute on each side and place it on a flat work surface.
- Divide the meat mixture, salsa, tomato and avocado on each tortilla and roll up to form into burritos. Slice into halves, transfer to a serving plate and serve immediately.

Seasoned Tilapia with Green Sauce

Preparation time: 10 minutes
Cooking time: 15 minutes
Serves: 4 to 6

Ingredients:

- 4 Tilapia fillets
- 1 tablespoon of onion powder
- 1 teaspoon of Spanish paprika
- 1 teaspoon of ground cumin
- Salt and crushed black pepper, to taste
- 2 tablespoons of ghee or olive oil

For the sauce:
- 2 ripe avocados, pitted and diced
- ½ cup of minced onions
- 2 jalapeno peppers, seeded and minced
- 3 organic limes, juiced
- 2 tablespoons of extra virgin olive oil
- 2 tablespoons of minced fresh cilantro leaves
- Salt and crushed black pepper, to taste

Directions:

1. Combine all sauce ingredients in a large bowl and set aside. Cover the bowl with plastic wrap and chill before using.
2. Preheat the oven to a temperature of 400°F. Lightly grease a baking pan with oil and set aside.
3. Combine all spices in a small bowl and rub evenly on both

sides of the tilapia. Place the tilapia on the prepared baking pan and drizzle with clarified butter on top of the tilapia. Bake it in the oven for 15 minutes or until the fish flakes easily with a fork and is cooked through. Remove from the oven and transfer to a serving plate.

4. Serve baked tilapia warm with green sauce.

Snacks & Appetizers

Golden Nutty Pecan Fat Bombs

Not only does this pecan fat bomb bars offer plenty of health benefits, but is also comes together with incredible ease and makes for a convenient protein snack that is nutty and aromatic at the same time!

Preparation Time: 5 Minutes

Cooking Time: 30 Minutes

Servings: Makes 12

Ingredients:

- 2 cups Pecans, halved
- ½ cup Shredded Coconut, unsweetened
- ¼ tsp. Liquid Stevia
- 1 cup Almond Flour
- ¼ cup Maple Syrup, homemade
- ½ cup Golden Flaxseed Meal
- ½ cup Coconut Oil

To make the maple syrup:

- ¾ cup Water
- 2 ¼ teaspoon Coconut Oil

- ¼ cup Erythritol, powdered
- ½ teaspoon Vanilla Extract
- 1 tablespoon Butter, unsalted
- ¼ teaspoon Xanthan Gum
- 2 teaspoon Maple Extract

Method of Preparation:

- To start with, bake the pecans on a baking sheet for about 5 to 8 minutes or until it becomes fragrant.

- After that, transfer the pecans into a plastic bag and then crush them with the help of a rolling pin.

- Next, take a medium sized bowl and then add the almond flour, shredded coconut and flax meal into it.

- Now, spoon in the crushed pecans and combine them well.

- Then, stir in the coconut oil, liquid stevia and maple syrup and mix them until you get a crumbly textured dough.

- Finally, place this dough on a baking sheet which is

lined with parchment paper and spread it evenly.

- Bake it for about 18 to 24 minutes or until the sides are becoming lightly browned.

- Remove the pan from the oven and allow it to cool.

- Once it is cooled, keep it in the refrigerator for another one minute so that it is set.

- **To make the maple syrup**, combine xanthan gum, butter and coconut oil in a medium sized bowl and microwave it for 30 to 50 seconds.

- Next, add the butter mixture with water and xantham gum along with stevia, maple extract and vanilla extract until they are well combined.

- Finally, microwave it again for another 40 seconds and allow it to cool.

Tip: If you are not able to use flaxseed meal, then you can use chia seeds, but 2/3 quantity.

Eat Fat and Get Thin, Fit, and Healthier Than Ever Before!

Nutritional Information:

- ➤ Calories – 303 kcal

- ➤ Fat – 30.5g

- ➤ Carbohydrates – 2gm

- ➤ Proteins – 4.9gm

Sunflower Seed Keto Crackers

These sunflower seeds crackers are extremely light and crispy while providing long lasting energy!

Preparation Time: 5 Minutes
Cooking Time: 45 Minutes
Servings: 6

Ingredients:
- 1 cup Sunflower Seeds, shelled
- ¼ cup Water
- ½ cup Parmesan Cheese, grated

Method of Preparation:
- To begin with, preheat the oven to 325-degree Fahrenheit.
- Next, place the sunflower seeds and the parmesan cheese in a food processor and process until it becomes a fine meal.
- To this, add water and then blend it again until you get a sticky dough.
- For the next step, take a cookie sheet which is lined

with parchment paper and then place the sticky dough and spread it on the cookie sheet.

- Now, place another parchment paper on top of the dough.

- After that, with the help of a rolling pen, flatten out the dough so that it becomes a thin sheet. (The more thinner it is, the more better it will be.)

- Then, remove the parchment paper that was kept on the top and then slice the sheet into smaller pieces to get the crackers by using a pizza cutter.

- Finally, bake them in the oven for 27 to 30 minutes or until it becomes lightly browned.

- Once it is done, peel the parchment paper from the bottom and allow it to cool for some time.

- Store it in dry containers.

Tip: To make it crunchier, you can add more sunflower seeds on top of the dough before it is kept for baking.

Nutritional Information:
- ➢ Calories – 150 kcal
- ➢ Fat – 12g
- ➢ Carbohydrates – 3.9g
- ➢ Proteins – 7.5
- ➢ Fiber – 2.1g

Eat Fat and Get Thin, Fit, and Healthier Than Ever Before!

Mushroom Black Pepper Chips

With your first bite, you will know why this very simple dish is the new favorite snack. The great texture of the fried mushrooms along with their deep earthy flavour makes it a refreshing snack.

Preparation Time: 15 Minutes

Cooking Time: 1 Hour

Servings:4

Ingredients:

- 10.6 oz Portobello Mushroom, preferably organic and sliced thinly
- Pinch of Black Pepper, freshly grounded
- 4 tablespoon Coconut Oil
- ½ teaspoon of Pink Himalayan Sea Salt

Method of Preparation:

1) To start with, preheat the oven to 300 degrees Fahrenheit.

2) After that, place the sliced mushroom on a baking sheet and then brush them with the coconut oil.

3) Next, sprinkle on top of these salt and pepper.

4) Next, bake them in the oven for 40 to 55 minutes or until they become brown and crispy. (While baking, rotate the baking sheet, so that all the slices are heated evenly.)

Tip: if you want them a bit spicy, you can add chilli powder or another spicy seasoning on top.

Nutritional Information:
- ➢ Calories – 169 kcal
- ➢ Fat -15.5gm
- ➢ Carbohydrates – 3.9gm
- ➢ Proteins – 3.2g
- ➢ Fiber – 2gm

Chicken Parmesan Keto Nuggets

Tender and juicy on the inside with a crunchy outside, this entrée embodies a scrumptious flavour which even the kids are sure to like.

Preparation Time: 15 Minutes

Cooking Time: 5 Minutes

Servings: 2

Ingredients:

- 4 oz. Chicken Breast, cooked
- 1 Egg, preferably organic and medium sized
- ½ Oz. Parmesan, grated
- ½ teaspoon Baking Powder
- 2 tablespoon Almond Flour
- Water, as required

Method of Preparation:

1) First heat your deep fryer to about 375 degrees.

2) Next, heat a skillet over medium-high heat and to this,

add coconut oil and cook the chicken until it is no longer pink in colour and is translucent.

3) Once it is cooked, cut the chicken pieces into cubes.

4) Now, combine almond flour, parmesan and baking powder in a medium-sized bowl and mix them well.

5) After that, stir in the egg to the bowl and whisk the mixture well until it is well incorporated.

6) Then, spoon in the chicken chops into this batter and combine until the chops are fully coated with the mixture.

7) Finally, fry them in the fryer for about 3 to 5 minutes or until they are golden brown in colour. (Make sure to stir them every minute so that the pieces won't stick to each other.)

8) Transfer them to a serving plate lined with a paper towel so as to remove the excess oil.

Tip: It pairs well with ranch dressing, but watch the sugar content!

Nutritional Information:

- ➤ Calories – 166 kcal
- ➤ Fat – 8gm
- ➤ Carbohydrates – 2gm
- ➤ Proteins – 23gm
- ➤ Fiber – 1gm

Eat Fat and Get Thin, Fit, and Healthier Than Ever Before!

Snacks and Appetizer Recipes

Feta-Stuffed Mushrooms

Serves: 4
Time: 17-20 minutes

These tasty little bites are the perfect appetizer for both low-carb and gluten-free dieters! Ingredients like bacon, feta, and spinach add flavor and nutrition, while seasonings like ground nutmeg and onion give the mushrooms depth.

Ingredients:

16 cleaned mushroom caps
8 slices chopped bacon
6 cups raw baby spinach
2 tablespoons butter
1 tablespoon almond flour
¼ cup chopped onion
⅓ cup crumbled feta cheese
¼ teaspoon ground nutmeg
Salt and pepper to taste

Directions:

1. Cook the bacon until crisp, and then add the onion and butter.
2. Cook for 3-5 minutes.
3. Remove the pan from heat and toss in the feta, almond flour, nutmeg, salt, and pepper.
4. Let the mixture cool.
5. Stuff the mushroom caps and arrange on a baking sheet.

6. Bake in a 375-degree oven for 15 minutes.
7. Serve right away!

Nutritional Info:

Total calories: 215
Carbs: 4
Fat: 16
Protein: 13
Fiber: 0

Pizza Bites

Serves: 6
Time: Less than 5 minutes

These pizza bites are so fast and pack in a lot of fat.
They're a great snack for between meals!

Ingredients:

14 slices of pepperoni
8 pitted black olives
4 ounces of cream cheese
2 tablespoons sun-dried tomato pesto
2 tablespoons fresh chopped basil
Salt and pepper to taste

Directions:

1. Dice the olives and pepperoni into little pieces.
2. Mix everything in a bowl.
3. Using very clean hands, form into six balls.
4. Eat!

Nutritional Info:

Total calories: 110
Carbs: 1.3
Fat: 10.5
Protein: 2.3
Fiber: 0

Cheesy Bacon Bites

Serves: 20
Time: Less than 10 minutes

If you need a pick-me-up during that long stretch between lunch and dinner, these cheese-filled, bacon-wrapped balls are just the ticket. The "ball" part is made from a dough that uses psyllium husk powder, which has been shown to improve digestion and make you feel full.

Ingredients:

10 bacon slices
8 ounces of mozzarella cheese
1 cup of olive oil
4 tablespoons melted butter
4 tablespoons almond flour
3 tablespoons psyllium husk powder
1 big egg
¼ teaspoon salt
¼ teaspoon black pepper
⅛ teaspoon onion powder

Directions:

1. Microwave half of the mozzarella cheese until it's melted.
2. Mix with the egg.
3. Microwave the butter until completely melted, then mix

with the egg/cheese.

4. Add the psyllium, almond flour, salt, black pepper, and onion powder.

5. Mix to form a dough.

6. Roll out the dough into a rectangle.

7. Fill with the remaining cheese and fold in half horizontally, and then vertically.

8. Crimp the edges with your fingers and form into another triangle.

9. Cut 20 squares.

10. Wrap the squares in half a piece of bacon and use toothpicks to secure.

11. Pour oil into a pan and heat to 350-375 degrees.

12. Fry the bites for 1-3 minutes, until bacon is cooked.

13. Lay on paper towels to absorb extra grease before eating.

Nutritional Info:

Total calories: 89
Carbs: .6
Fat: 7.2
Protein: 5
Fiber: 1.2

Broccoli-Cheddar Biscuits

Serves: 12
Time: 20 minutes

Biscuits on a keto diet? Yes, indeed, when you use almond flour. The result is cheesy, broccoli-studded biscuits that are spiced with paprika, garlic powder, and a little apple cider vinegar.

Ingredients:

4 cups raw broccoli florets
2 cups cheddar cheese
1 ½ cup almond flour
¼ cup coconut oil
2 big eggs
1 teaspoon paprika
1 teaspoon garlic powder
1 teaspoon salt
½ teaspoon black pepper
½ teaspoon apple cider vinegar
½ teaspoon baking soda

Directions:

1. Preheat your oven to 375-degrees.
2. Chop up the broccoli in a food processor.
3. Mix the flour with the spices.
4. Add the vinegar, melted coconut oil, and eggs.

5. Mix to form a dough.

6. Add the cheese and broccoli, and mix well.

7. Form 12 biscuits and put them on a greased cookie sheet.

8. Bake for 12-15 minutes.

9. At this point, you should remove them from the oven and shape them to look more like biscuits.

10. Bake for another 5 minutes.

11. Turn the oven to broil and leave under the broiler for 4-5 minutes.

12. Let the biscuits cool for a few minutes before removing them and letting them cool another 10 minutes more on a plate.

Nutritional Info:

Total calories: 163
Carbs: 2
Fat: 14.3
Protein: 6.8
Fiber: 1.8

Chai Spice Mug Cake

Serves: 1
Time: About 2 minutes

This is probably the quickest dessert you could make. It's like a winter's day bundled up by a fire. All it takes is a microwave, a mug, and the following ingredients.

Ingredients:

1 big room-temperature egg
2 tablespoons almond flour
2 tablespoons butter
1 tablespoon Erythritol
7 drops of stevia
½ teaspoon baking powder
2 tablespoons almond flour
¼ teaspoon ground ginger
¼ teaspoon cinnamon
¼ teaspoon cardamom
¼ teaspoon vanilla
¼ teaspoon ground clove

Directions:

1. Mix everything together in a large mug.
2. Microwave on high for 70 seconds.
3. To remove the cake, turn the cup upside down and tap it lightly.
4. If you want, top with whipped cream and more cinnamon.

Nutritional Info:

Total calories: 439
Carbs: 4
Fat: 42
Protein: 12
Fiber: 3

Maple-Pecan Bars

Serves: 12
Time: 1 hour, 30 minutes (overnight for the maple syrup)

These sweet, nutty bars are a great source of fat and can be eaten any time of the day as a snack. You don't *need* to toast the pecans beforehand, but the toasting adds a lot of good flavor. To keep this recipe keto-friendly, you make your own no-carb maple syrup substitute that's really easy.

Ingredients:

2 cups of pecan halves
1 cup almond flour
½ cup of golden flaxseed meal (Bob's Red Mill is a good brand)
½ cup coconut oil
½ cup unsweetened, shredded coconut
¼ cup no-carb "maple syrup"
¼ teaspoon liquid stevia

"Maple Syrup" ingredients

3 cups water
2 tablespoons maple flavor
5 drops lemon flavor
2 cups stevia in the raw
1 teaspoon xanthan gum
⅛ teaspoon salt

Directions:

1. To make the syrup, mix 2 cups of water and both

flavorings in a big bowl.
2. In a separate bowl, whisk the stevia, salt, and xanthan gum together.
3. Slowly whisk the dry ingredients into the water.
4. When mixed well, whisk again (vigorously) with the last cup of water.
5. Cover with plastic wrap and store in the fridge overnight.
6. Puree until totally smooth.
7. Store tightly in jars and keep in the fridge.
8. Now, let's make the actual maple-pecan bars.
9. Toast the pecans on a cookie sheet for 6-8 minutes in a 350-degree oven.
10. Crush.
11. Mix all the dry ingredients together, including the toasted pecans.
12. Add the wet ingredients and mix until you get a crumbly-dough consistency.
13. With your hands, press down into a 11x7-inch casserole dish and bake at 350-degrees for 20-25 minutes.
14. Let the bars cool completely before storing in the fridge for *at least* 1 hour.
15. Cut into bars.

Nutritional Info:

Total calories: 303
Carbs: 2
Fat: 30.5
Protein: 4.9
Fiber: <1

Dessert Recipes

Coconut Cocoa Candy

You will be amazed at how much flavour these coconut oil candies have! They are incredibly easy to make, they taste great and are best to satisfy your evening sugar cravings!

Preparation Time: 5 Minutes

Cooking Time: 1-hour plus to cool

Servings: Makes 18 candies

Ingredients:

- 1 cup Virgin Coconut Oil, cold pressed and softened

- 1 teaspoon Vanilla Extract

- 1 to 2 tablespoon Swerve

- ½ tsp Celtic Sea Salt

- 2 to 4 tablespoon Cocoa powder, unsweetened and organic

- 2 tablespoon Almond Butter

Method of Preparation:

- To begin with, place the virgin coconut oil, cocoa

powder, salt, vanilla extract, almond butter and swerve in a food processor and then process them until it becomes a smooth liquid.

- Next, drop the coconut oil mixture into a baking sheet lined with parchment paper.

- Finally, refrigerate them by keeping it in the fridge until it becomes solid. Store them in a dry container for later use.

Tip: Instead of almond butter it is also possible to use any other nut butter. Similarly, you can use unsweetened desiccated coconut to sprinkle on top of these candies.

Nutritional Information:
- ➢ Calories – 210 kcal
- ➢ Fat – 22gm
- ➢ Carbohydrates – 1.24gm
- ➢ Fiber – 1gm

Lone Star Keto Cake

Would you be intrested in a recipe that you can incorporate into your diet to help with weight loss?Then, make this this dessert which is every peanut butter lovers dream dessert!

Preparation Time: 15 Minutes
Cooking Time: 1 Hour + 1 Hour cooling time
Servings: Serves 20
Ingredients:

- 2 cups Almond flour

- ½ cup Butter, preferably organic

- ¼ cup Cocoa powder

- 1/3 cup Coconut flour

- 3 Eggs, preferably large and farm fed

- 1/3 cup Whey Protein powder, unflavored

- 1 tablespoon Baking powder

- ½ teaspoon Sea Salt

- ¼ cup Water

- ¼ cup Heavy Cream

- ½ cup Water

- 1 teaspoon Vanilla Extract

To make the frosting:

- ¼ tsp Xanthan gum

- ½ cup Butter

- 1 ½ cups powdered Swerve Sweetener
- ¼ cup Cocoa powder
- ¾ cup Pecans, coarsely chopped
- ¼ cup Cream
- ¼ cup Water
- 1 teaspoon Vanilla Extract

Method of Preparation:

1) To begin with, preheat the oven to 325 degrees Fahrenheit.

2) After that, combine almond flour, baking powder, coconut flour, protein powder and salt in a large sized bowl until they are well incorporated. (Make sure to ensure that there are no clumps in it.)

3) Next, take a non-stick pan and heat it over medium heat.

4) Now, add the butter, cocoa powder and water into it and stir it well until the butter is melted and the

mixture starts boiling.

5) Spoon this cocoa mixture also into the mixing bowl and stir them together.

6) Then, add the eggs, heavy cream, water and vanilla extract to the mixing bowl and combine until it is properly combined.

7) Finally, pour the batter into a baking sheet lined with buttered parchment paper and bake it in the oven for 16 to 21 minutes or until a toothpick inserted in the centre comes clean.

8) To make the frosting, take another non stick pan of medium size and stir in butter, cream, cocoa powder and water and combine it well.

9) Bring the mixture to a simmer and then spoon in the vanilla extract and mix it well.

10)   Once it mixed well, add the swerve gradually half a cup at a time and stir it.

11)   Finally, stir in the xanthum gum into it until the mixture becomes a smooth batter.

12)   Pour this mixture over the warm cake and then top the cake with the chopped pecans.

13)   Allow the cake to cool so that the frosting gets set. Enjoy the delicious cake.

Tip: If you are not able to use almond flour, you can try using sunflower seeds flour.

Nutritional Information:

> ➢   Calorie – 230 kcal
> ➢   Fat – 20.32g
> ➢   Carbohydrates – 2.8gm
> ➢   Proteins – 5.76g
> ➢   Fiber – 3.06g

Amazing Avocado Sorbet

Are you looking for different ways to include avocado into your diets? Then this rich and completlely satisfying sorbet would be the perfect way while being totally sugarless and low in carbohydrates!

Preparation Time: 5 Minutes

Cooking Time: 15 Minutes

Servings: 5

Ingredients:

- 2 cups Almond Milk, unsweetened
- 1 teaspoon Mango Extract
- 2 ripe Avocados
- ½ tsp Celtic Sea Salt
- 2 tablespoon Lime juice
- ¾ cup Swerve sweetener (optional)

Method of Preparation:

1) To begin with, place the almond milk, avocados, mango extract, swerve (optional), lime juice and sea salt

together in a food processor and blend until it becomes a smooth puree.

2) Next, transfer the puree to the chilled container of the ice cream machine.

3) Follow the instructions given by the manufacturers of the ice cream machine and make the ice cream.

4) Once the ice cream is made, transfer the contents to a container and place it in the freezer.

Tip: If after tasting the ice cream, the sweetness doesn't seem correct, then you can add more and freeze it again as it will not be affected by this process.

Nutritional Information:

- ➤ Calories – 146 kcal
- ➤ Fat – 13.2gm
- ➤ Carbohydrates – 2.4gm
- ➤ Protein – 2gm
- ➤ Fiber – 5.8gm

Low Carb Strawberry Pecan Cheesecake

Have one bite of this low carb strawberry cheesecake and it would surely be an instant, love at first sight with this cheesecake since it comes with a great texture and creamy flavour. Don't miss a chance to have this ultimate low carb dessert.

Preparation Time: 30 Minutes
Cooking Time: 90 Minutes
Servings: 8

Ingredients:

To make the crust

- ¾ Cup Pecans
- 4 tablespoon Butter, preferably organic
- ¾ Cup Almond Flour
- 2 tablespoon Splenda

To make the filling:

- 1½ lbs Cream Cheese
- ¼ cup Sour Cream
- 4 Eggs, preferably medium and organic

- 9 organic Strawberries, sliced
- ½ tablespoon Liquid Vanilla
- 1 cup Splenda
- ½ tablespoon Lemon Juice

Method of Preparation:

1) To begin with, preheat the oven to 400-degree Fahrenheit.

2) After that, place the pecan in a plastic bag and crush them by using a rolling pin.

3) Next, take a saucepan and heat it over medium heat.

4) To this, add the butter, almond flour, Splenda and crushed pecans and combine them well to make the dough for the crust.

5) Transfer the crust into a baking pan greased with butter and spread it out evenly.

6) Now, bake it in the oven for about 5 to 7 minutes or until it is browned.

7) To make the filling, take a standing mixer, and place the cream cheese, eggs, lemon juice, sour cream, Splenda and liquid vanilla in it.

8) Then, blend them well until it becomes a smooth batter. Transfer the liquid mixture into the baking pan and spread them evenly.

9) Place the strawberries onto the side and top of the crust.

10)   Finally, bake the cheesecake at 250 degrees Fahrenheit and cook for about one hour to 90 minutes until it has been set.

11)   Transfer the cake to the working station and allow it to be cooled.

12)   Once cooled, place it in the refrigerator.

Tip: When serving, top it with the whipped cream.

Eat Fat and Get Thin, Fit, and Healthier Than Ever Before!

Nutritional Information:

- ➤ Calories – 535 kcal
- ➤ Fat – 49gm
- ➤ Carbohydrates – 9gm
- ➤ Proteins – 13gm
- ➤ Fiber – 2gm

Chocolate Avocado Keto Brownies

If you are looking for holiday desserts that are low in carbs, then do try these after dinner dessert for sure. They are rich while being healthy.

Preparation Time: 15 Minutes
Cooking Time: 25 Minutes
Servings: Makes 16

Ingredients:
- 3.5 oz dark chocolate, broken
- 1 Avocado, ripe and preferably large
- ¼ cup Butter
- ¼ cup Coconut flour
- 3 Eggs, preferably large and organic
- ¼ tsp Pink Himalayan salt
- ¾ cup powdered Erythritol
- ¼ cup coconut milk
- 1 ½ cups Almond flour
- 2 tsp Baking powder

- ½ cup Cacao powder, unsweetened

Method of Preparation:

1) To start with, preheat the oven to 350 degrees Fahrenheit.

2) After that, take a bowl and place it in a thick bottomed pan filled half-way with water.

3) Then, put the dark chocolate pieces in the bowl and then heat the pan over medium heat.Bring the water to a boil and then lower the heat.

4) Next, stir in the butter to the bowl and melt it while stirring occasionally.

5) In the meantime, place the eggs in the bowl of the standing mixer and to this add the Erythritol and combine until soft peaks form.

6) Now, add the scooped avocado flesh and the coconut milk into a blender and blend until it becomes a smooth puree.

7) Then, pour the avocado puree into the egg mixture and whisk them until they are well combined.

8) At this point, spoon in the chocolate mixture and mix them again until they are properly mixed.

9) Once they are combined well, take another bowl and place the almond flour, baking powder, coconut flour and salt and blend them well.

10)   Finally, mix the almond mixture into the wet mixture and blend them well.

11)   Transfer the mixture into a baking pan lined with parchment paper. Flatten it with a spatula.

12)   Bake it in the oven for about 18 to 25 minutes or until it is set.

13)   Place the brownie outside for a while until it is cooled. Once cooled, cut into smaller pieces.

Tip: it pairs well with heavy whipped cream.

Nutritional Information:

- ➢ Calories – 169 kcal
- ➢ Fat – 14.8gm
- ➢ Carbohydrates – 3.8gm
- ➢ Proteins – 5.1g
- ➢ Fiber – 3.5g

Eat Fat and Get Thin, Fit, and Healthier Than Ever Before!

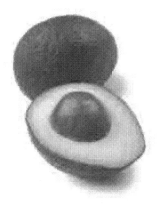

Part 3: 21 Day Meal Plan

Week 1

DAY	Breakfast	Lunch	Dinner
1	Spinach Omelet and Avocado 134	Turkey Breast Avocado Sandwich 140	Walnut-Crusted Baked Salmon Fillets 72
2	Chicken Sausage Breakfast Pie 42	Sliced Chicken Burrito 154	Spice-Rubbed Chicken with Avocado Salsa 144
3	Fast and Cheesy Jalapeno Cheddar Waffles 46	Smoked Salmon Frittata with Avocado 132	Nacho Chicken Casserole 74
4	Chorizo Breakfast Casserole 52	Broccoli-Cheddar Biscuits 178	Baked Salmon with Avocado Salsa 150
5	Crustless Two Cheese Quiche 56	Clam Chowder 94	Crispy Baked Chicken Wings 76
6	Keto Breakfast Protein Smoothie 60	Taco-Spiced Turkey Burrito 136	Seasoned Tilapia with Green Sauce 156
7	Jalapeno-Popper Cups 44	Broccoli-Chicken Zucchini Boats 62	Fresh Snapper Ceviche 146

Week 2

DAY	Breakfast	Lunch	Dinner
8	Easiest Egg-Drop Soup 64	Sliced Chicken Burrito 154	Mexican Benedict Chipotle Sauce 138
9	Broccoli-Cheddar Biscuits 178	Baked Salmon with Avocado Salsa 150	Greek Meatballs with Avocado Tzatziki Sauce 148
10	Green Eggs and Butter 48	Easiest Egg-Drop Soup 64	Sliced Chicken Burrito 154
11	Chicken Sausage Breakfast Pie 42	Turkey Breast Avocado Sandwich 140	Chicken Parmesan 78
12	Chorizo Breakfast Casserole 52	Salmon, Avocado and Cucumber Green Salad 142	Korean Beef-Stuffed Peppers 80
13	Spinach Omelet and Avocado 134	Golden Nutty Pecan Fat Bombs 158	Vegan Tofu Tacos 152
14	Crustless Two Cheese Quiche 56	Portobello Pizzas 66	Easy Paprika Chicken 82

Week 3

D A Y	Breakfast	Lunch	Dinner
1 5	Keto Breakfast Protein Smoothie 60	Baked Salmon with Avocado Salsa 150	Cucumber Sushi Rolls 88
1 6	Breakfast Mug Cake 40	Pork Chops w/ a Cumin Crust 68	Spectacular Seafood and Bacon 128_
1 7	Green Eggs and Butter 48	Feta-Stuffed Mushrooms 172	Taco-Spiced Turkey Burrito 136
1 8	Chicken Sausage Breakfast Pie 42	Spice-Rubbed Chicken with Avocado Salsa 144	Baked Squash and Beef Lasagna 120
1 9	Easiest Egg-Drop Soup 64	Oven-Baked Sweet + Sour Chicken 70	Nutty Almond Stromboli 112
2 0	Jalapeno-Popper Cups 44	Smoked Salmon Frittata with Avocado 132	Sunflower-Butter Pork Kabobs 108
2 1	Keto Breakfast Protein Smoothie 60	Fresh Snapper Ceviche 146	Salmon, Avocado and Cucumber Green Salad 142

Eat Fat and Get Thin, Fit, and Healthier Than Ever Before!

Made in the USA
Lexington, KY
07 August 2016